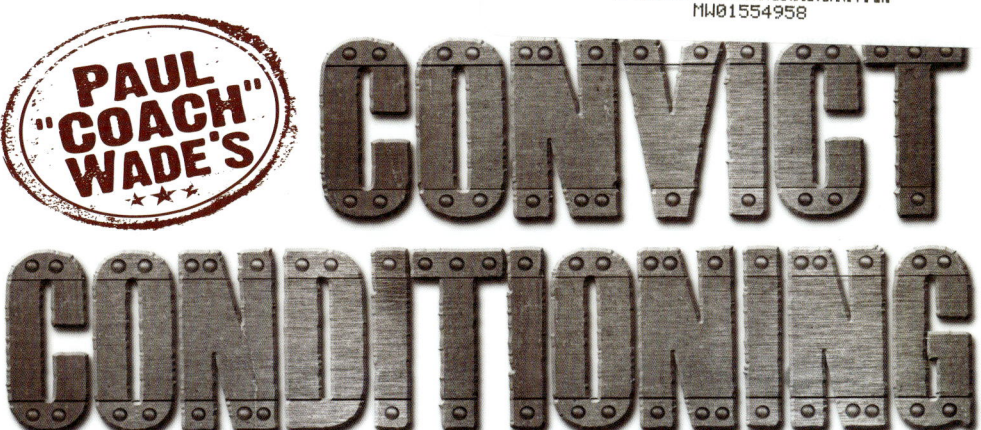

ULTIMATE BODYWEIGHT TRAINING LOG

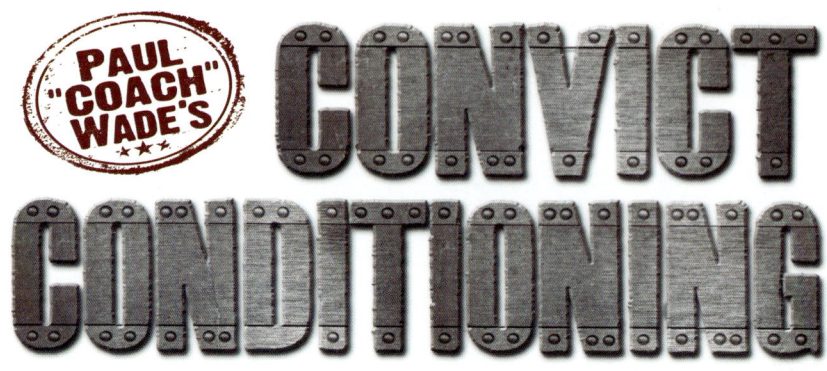

Ultimate Bodyweight
Training Log

Copyright ©2012 Paul "Coach" Wade
All rights under International and Pan-American Copyright conventions.

Published in the United States by:
Dragon Door Publications, Inc
5 East County Rd B, #3 • Little Canada, MN 55117
Tel: (651) 487-2180 • Fax: (651) 487-3954
Credit card orders: 1-800-899-5111
Email: support@dragondoor.com • Website: www.dragondoor.com

This edition first published in December, 2012
ISBN 10: 0-938045-98-9   ISBN 13: 978-0-938045-98-4

No part of this book may be reproduced in any form or by any means without the prior written consent of the Publisher, excepting brief quotes used in reviews.

Printed in China

Book design, and cover by Derek Brigham
Website www.dbrigham.com • Tel/Fax: (763) 208-3069 • Email: bigd@dbrigham.com

Photography by Marc Blondin Photography

DISCLAIMER
The author and publisher of this material are not responsible in any manner whatsoever for any injury that may occur through following the instructions contained in this material. The activities, physical and otherwise, described herein for informational purposes only, may be too strenuous or dangerous for some people and the reader(s) should consult a
physician before engaging in them.

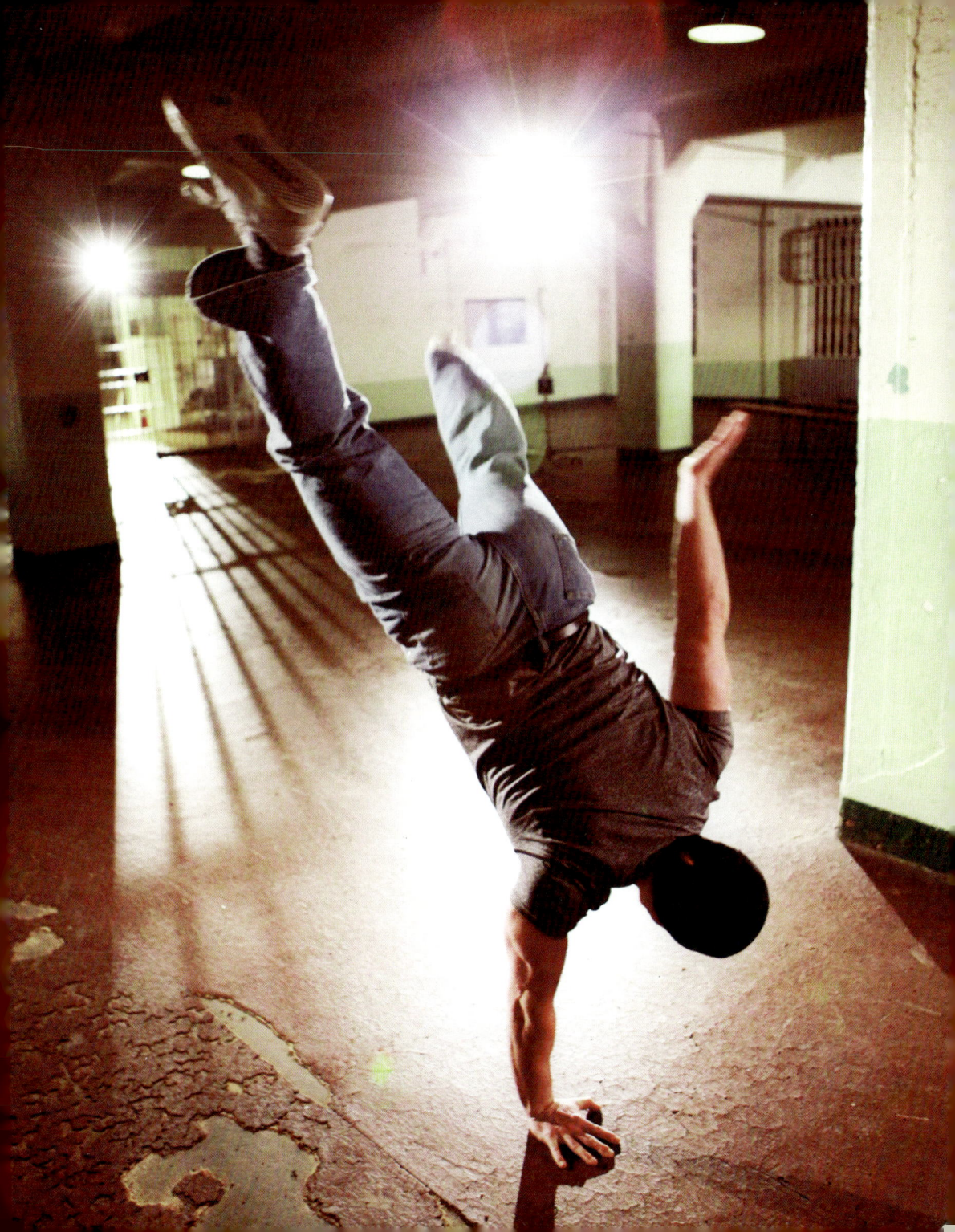

DISCLAIMER!

Fitness and strength are meaningless qualities without *health*. With correct training, these three benefits should naturally proceed hand-in-hand. In this book, every effort has been made to convey the importance of safe training technique, but despite this all individual trainees are different and needs will vary. Proceed with caution, and at your own risk. Your body is your own responsibility-look after it. All medical experts agree that you should consult your physician before initiating a training program. Be safe!

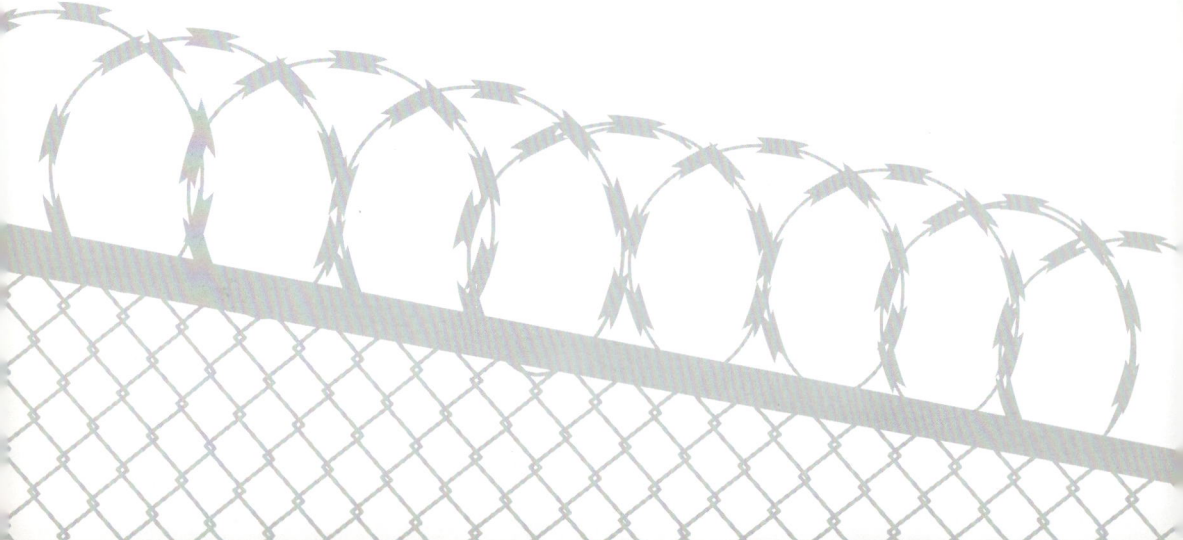

TABLE OF CONTENTS

PART I: INFO AND WORKOUTS

Intro	1
Progressive Calisthenics	3
Goals and Goal-Setting	7
Convict Conditioning: The Workouts	11
How to Use This Log	19

PART II: LOG ENTRIES

Training Journal	24

PART III: CHARTS & CHECKLISTS

Calisthenics Anatomy	248
Personal Records	250
Six Month Weight Stats	252
CC Progression Tables	254
Notes	260

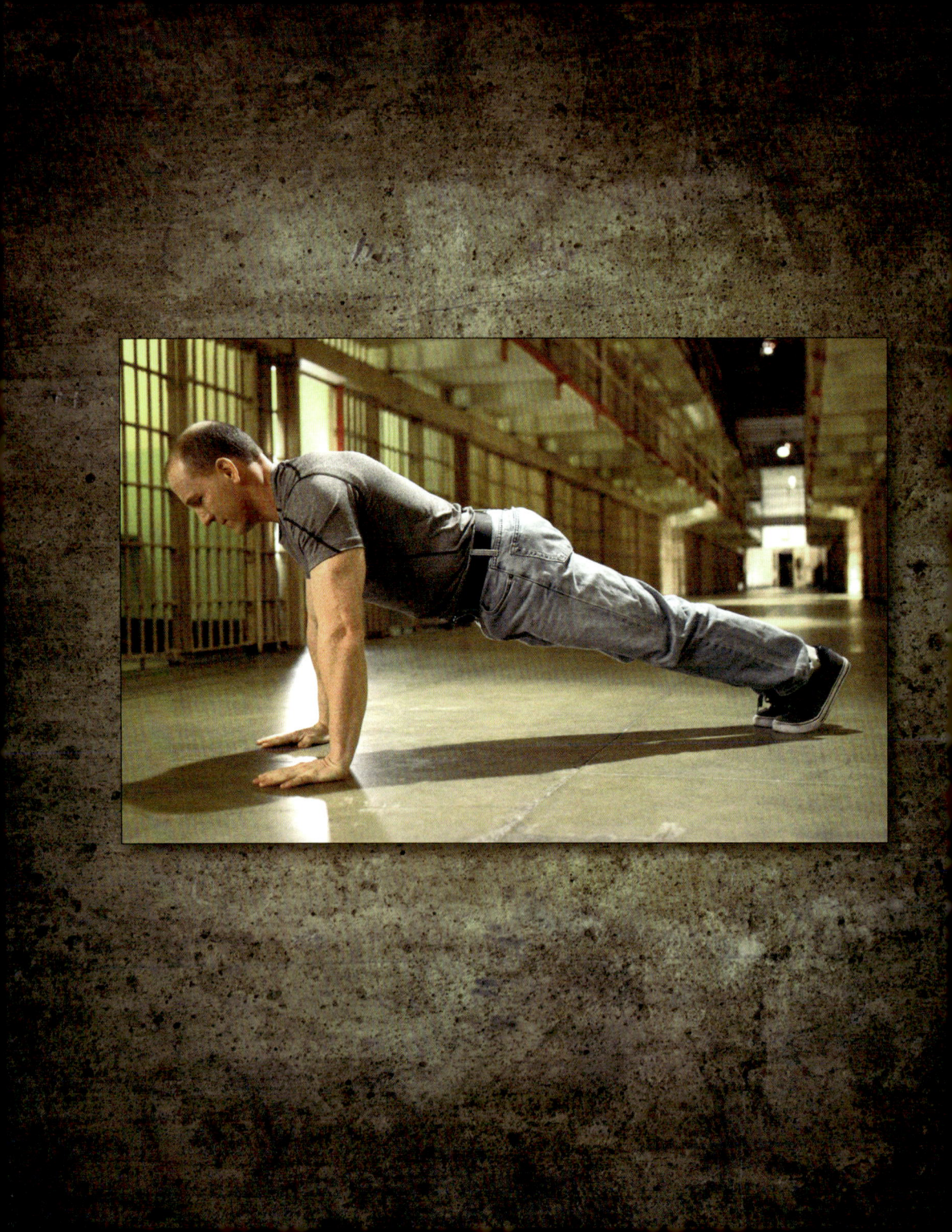

PART I:
Info & Workouts

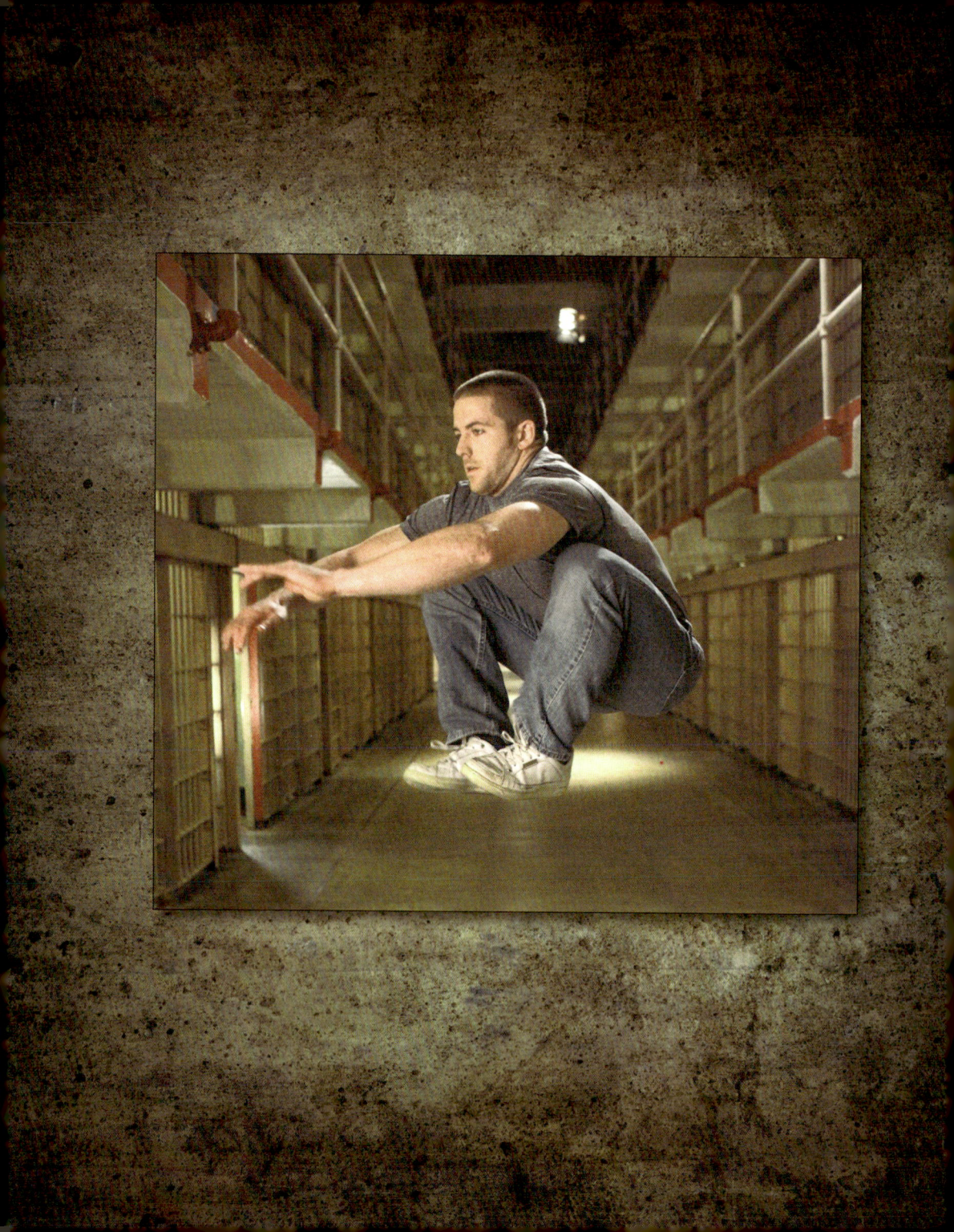

INTRO

When it comes to serious training, you keep a log or you fail. The sooner you learn this, the better.

During the years I was mastering bodyweight training in jail, I met a great many potentially *phenomenal* athletes who failed to reach *anywhere near* their maximum ability because they never kept a record of their workouts. A lot of these guys just "kinda" or "sorta" remembered how their last couple of training sessions went—and hardly any had any medium or long-term training goals. Many of them were very "instinctive" trainers, who just worked out until they felt tired, or until it was time for a smoke. As a result they never really hit that target zone, that golden *window of opportunity* they needed to progress in their training, even by fractions, week-by-week. So most of these guys (unless they were on steroids) just kept looking the same, year-in, year-out.

Make no mistake: a workout journal is a very powerful, widely underestimated tool for unlocking your physical potential. That's why, when I wrote ***Convict Conditioning***, I made damn sure there was a detailed section inside that book on the importance of keeping a solid training journal. ***Convict Conditioning*** went on to become one of the best-selling bodyweight training books of all time (my bookie thanks you all), but I discovered later that a lot of my readers didn't take my advice on keeping a training log. Some told me they couldn't be assed structuring a log entry after an exhausting, kick-ass workout; some were honest and said they felt it was a pain in the butt to figure out all that writing.

There were other reasons, too. More than a few of my students told me they had tried buying off-the-shelf training logs, but discovered that they were simply cookie-cutter templates meant for the average weight-using gym-goer, rather than serious bodyweight athletes—sadly they just weren't suitable for the bodyweight guys and gals. After looking through a bunch of these logs, I realized this was true—there really was no ready-structured training journal suitable for my bodyweight students.

"Okay," I thought, "dammit. I'll write one for ya."

And here it is.

About this log

This book is the first ever training log designed specifically for bodyweight athletes. Other logs are structured to contain sections where you detail the amount of weight you used, the type of equipment or machine you worked out on, even what your heart-rate was and what vitamins you took today. You won't find any of this distracting crap in this log. It's a log for pure, unadulterated, hardcore bodyweight training. As such, it can be used for *any* kind of bodyweight program you wish to use—not just Convict Conditioning.

I'll begin this log with a few ideas on the best "whys and hows" about keeping a training log. Then I'll share with you six classic Convict Conditioning programs, and guide you on when to use each one. There's also a section to record your goals and PRs, as well as some help on approaching these aspects of training. Since your weight is a crucial aspect of calisthenics, this log contains an easy-to-use six month bodyweight chart for you to fill in. At the end of the book, I've included some at-a-glance charts to help you progress with your bodyweight skills.

The meat of any training log is the daily log entries. This log contains more than a hundred potential entries—which, depending on what routine you use, may be up to a full year of workouts: probably closer to six months or more for the average athlete. Rather than just being a stock template, every log page is paired with advanced training tips, ideas and notes (some from my own training journals) to keep you on the straight and narrow. Each daily entry is also accompanied by (previously unseen) bodyweight training photo—many straight from "The Rock", Alcatraz penitentiary. If that doesn't keep those motivational fires burning, nothing will!

Paul "Coach" Wade

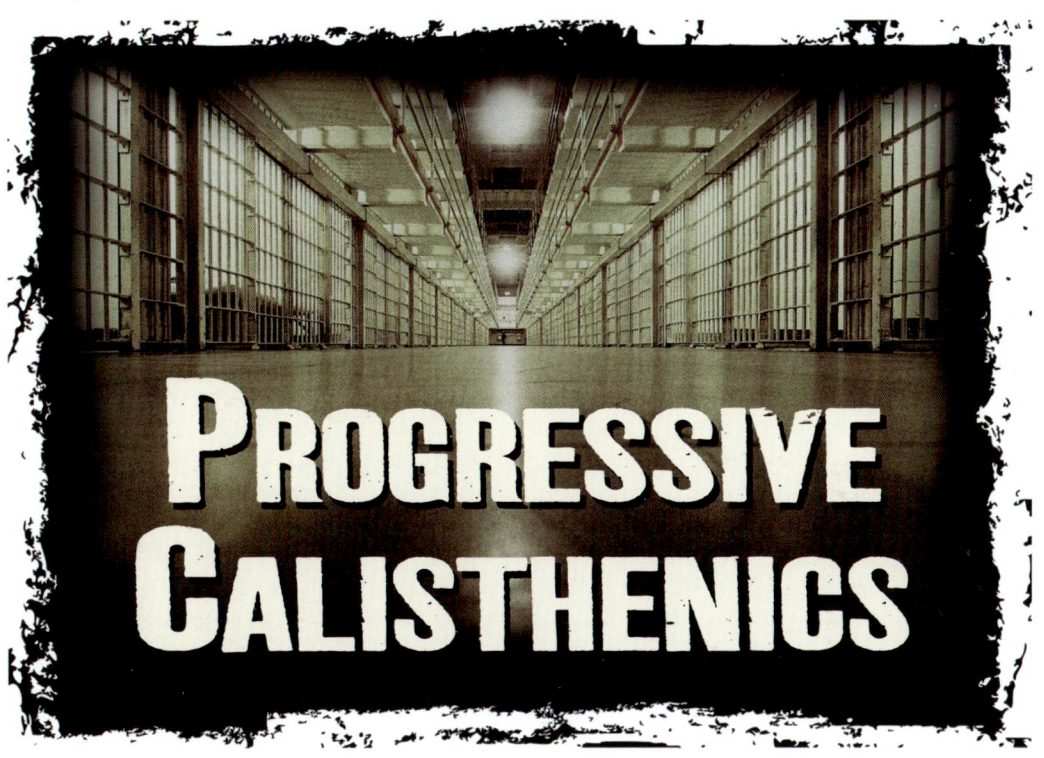

Progressive Calisthenics

Bodyweight training is about more than pushups and sit-ups. As convicts, gymnasts and martial artists have known for centuries, bodyweight training can be used to achieve peak human strength, power and muscularity.

To use bodyweight training this way, you simply apply the same principle of *progression* used in weight-training. In weight-training, you begin a lift using a certain weight; over time you get stronger, and can handle the weight better. Your form improves; the weight doesn't exhaust you so much; you add reps. When you can perform a target number of reps, you increase the weight, and the cycle repeats itself. You can follow the exact same principle with bodyweight training, but when you reach your target reps, you don't add *weight*—you move to a *slightly harder version of the exercise*. This method is called *progressive calisthenics*, and it leads you from kneeling pushups to one-arm pushups, from knee tucks to strict hanging leg raises, from bodyweight squats to one-leg squats, from clutch hangs to the human flag, from horizontal rows to one-arm pullups, and so on.

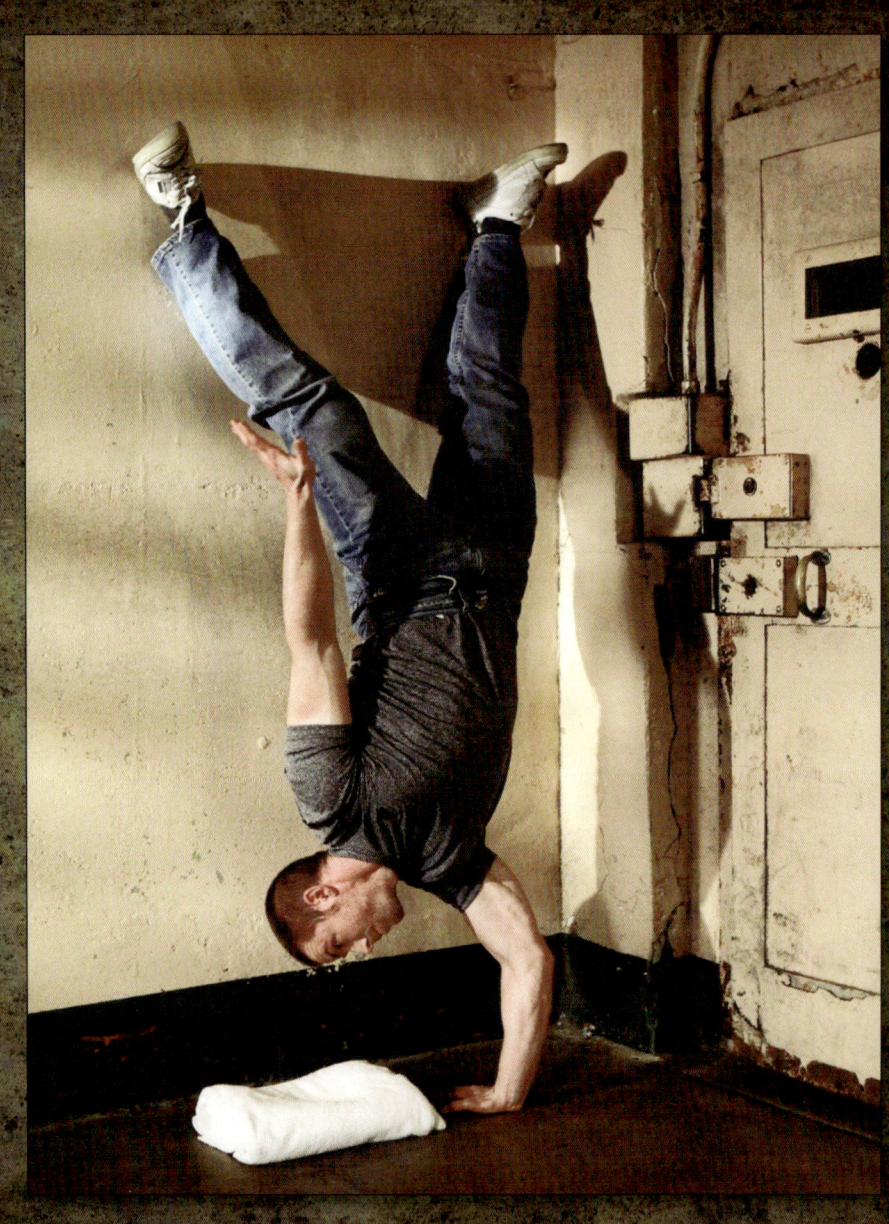

This idea sounds simple (and it is), but the key lies in knowing how and when to progress from one exercise to the next, and which exercise to progress to. The books *Convict Conditioning* and *Convict Conditioning 2* and the *Convict Conditioning DVD Series* provide a complete breakdown of these exercise chains, from the easiest bodyweight exercises to the hardest versions for super-advanced athletes. You should refer to those resources for complete information (like technical descriptions), but for reference sake this training log contains a full series of Convict Conditioning progression charts, starting on page 254.

Why you need a training log

If making progress in training is so simple, why do so few wannabe athletes ever achieve a good level of strength and muscle—let alone a *great* level?

The answer is that few trainees take advantage of the *windows of opportunity* their training presents to them. You see, when you work out, your body adapts to cope with the stress, but it only adapts a tiny little bit; this is especially true once you get beyond the beginner stages of training. Improvements are small—maybe you add a rep here; you improve your form there; you increase your recovery time somewhere else. Over months and years, however, these small increases eventually add up to very big increases. This is how seemingly "inhuman" athletes double and triple their strength, add inches of solid muscle, and transform themselves into superior physical beings.

Sadly, since most trainees aren't paying attention to those tiny changes, they never build on them the way they should. These little weekly changes are actually *windows of opportunity*. If you could increase your strength by just 1% every week, you could more than double your strength in just two years. But most trainees never get anywhere close to doubling their strength, because they aren't keeping track of their training accurately. They fail to recognize that 1% adaptation—the rep here, the improved form there. If you miss these *little* improvements, how can you build on them to make *big* improvements?

1% is actually a pretty small target to hit. When you rely on memory, instinct or feeling—as so many trainers do—to hit this target, it becomes very *fuzzy*. (Which is the last thing you want from small target, right?) Writing your progress down in a log makes this small target clear and easy to see. It makes it quantifiable. Athletes who begin writing simple log entries of their workouts find they suddenly know what they need to do to progress every single time they work out. They never miss that tiny 1%.

Keeping a log doesn't just help you see when you are making progress. It acts as an early warning system to let you know when you are *not* making progress. By checking their log to look at their progress levels over the short-term, athletes can quickly discover whether their training program is working or not. This is the kind of knowledge that helps individuals learn what types of training or techniques really work for their bodies—rather than just guessing at what "feels" right. It's this kind of knowledge that separates truly great athletes from the also-rans.

A log makes life easier!

The idea of training efficiency brings me to another point. A lot of athletes see writing in a training log as a *drag*; a drain on time and energy. This is a misconception—a log will *save* you time and mental energy in the long run. An endless list of studies show that people who actually *write down* their goals and progress become much higher achievers; quicker, and with less effort. Why is this? Simply because when your targets and actions are set down in black-and-white, you don't have to waste so much goddam time and energy thinking or talking about them. The human memory is notoriously shaky and deceptive compared to pen and ink anyway—and with a training log, you'll never have to struggle to remember where you're at. Best of all, a simple training log could save you months—or even years—of wasted effort on substandard routines.

With the *Convict Conditioning Ultimate Bodyweight Training Log*, there are no excuses. You don't even have to structure an entry—just fill in the blank sections with your training, and you're done.

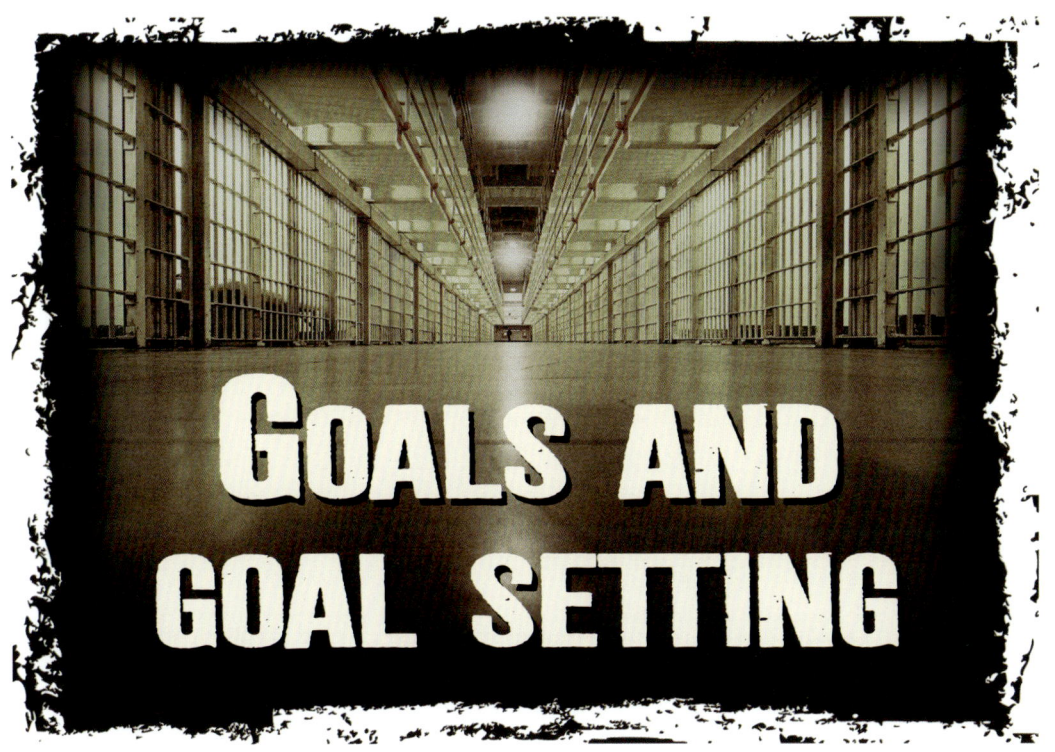

Goals and Goal Setting

A workout log is an ideal place to write down some training goals. Page nine has been left clear for you to set down any training goals you want. These can be *long-term* (years), *medium-term* (months) or even *short-term* (weeks and days)—whatever fires your imagination. Some examples of realistic goals to meet over the next 100+ workouts might be:

- Graduating two steps in an upper-body exercise
  (e.g., going from regular *full pullups* to *uneven pullups*);
- Graduating two steps in a lower-body exercise
  (e.g., going from *uneven squats* to *assisted one-leg squats*);

- Adding some muscle size (e.g., putting an inch on your guns);
- Improving your conditioning (e.g., doubling your exercises, doubling your sets, tripling your reps, halving your rest time, etc.);
- Adding something new to your training routine (e.g., adding some explosive variants, mobility work, grip work, into your workouts);
- Dropping some weight to help your calisthenics progress (e.g., losing 15 pounds).

Don't set too many goals at any one time; the more you set, the less likely you'll meet them all. Two or three serious goals are better than six or seven half-assed ones. Effort, like peanut butter and jelly, can be spread too thinly.

Be *specific* when you write your goals. (If your goals aren't specific, it's harder to meet them.) For example, don't write: *I want to be able to do more bodyweight squats*; write: *I want to be able to perform 100 reps of bodyweight squats in a single set*. Also, give each goal a specific time limit; for example: *I want to be able to perform 100 reps of bodyweight squats in a single set by June this year*.

Lastly, try not to get obsessed with meeting your goals. Drive is great, but remember that your goals exist for *you*—you don't exist for *them*. You can change them if you need to. If life throws you a curveball and you gotta adapt, then adapt—that's what survivors do.

EXISTING LEVEL

CURRENT DATE: _____
_____
_____
_____

CURRENT DATE: _____
_____
_____
_____

CURRENT DATE: _____
_____
_____
_____

CURRENT DATE: _____
_____
_____
_____

FUTURE GOAL

TARGET DATE: _____
_____
_____
_____

TARGET DATE: _____
_____
_____
_____

TARGET DATE: _____
_____
_____
_____

TARGET DATE: _____
_____
_____
_____

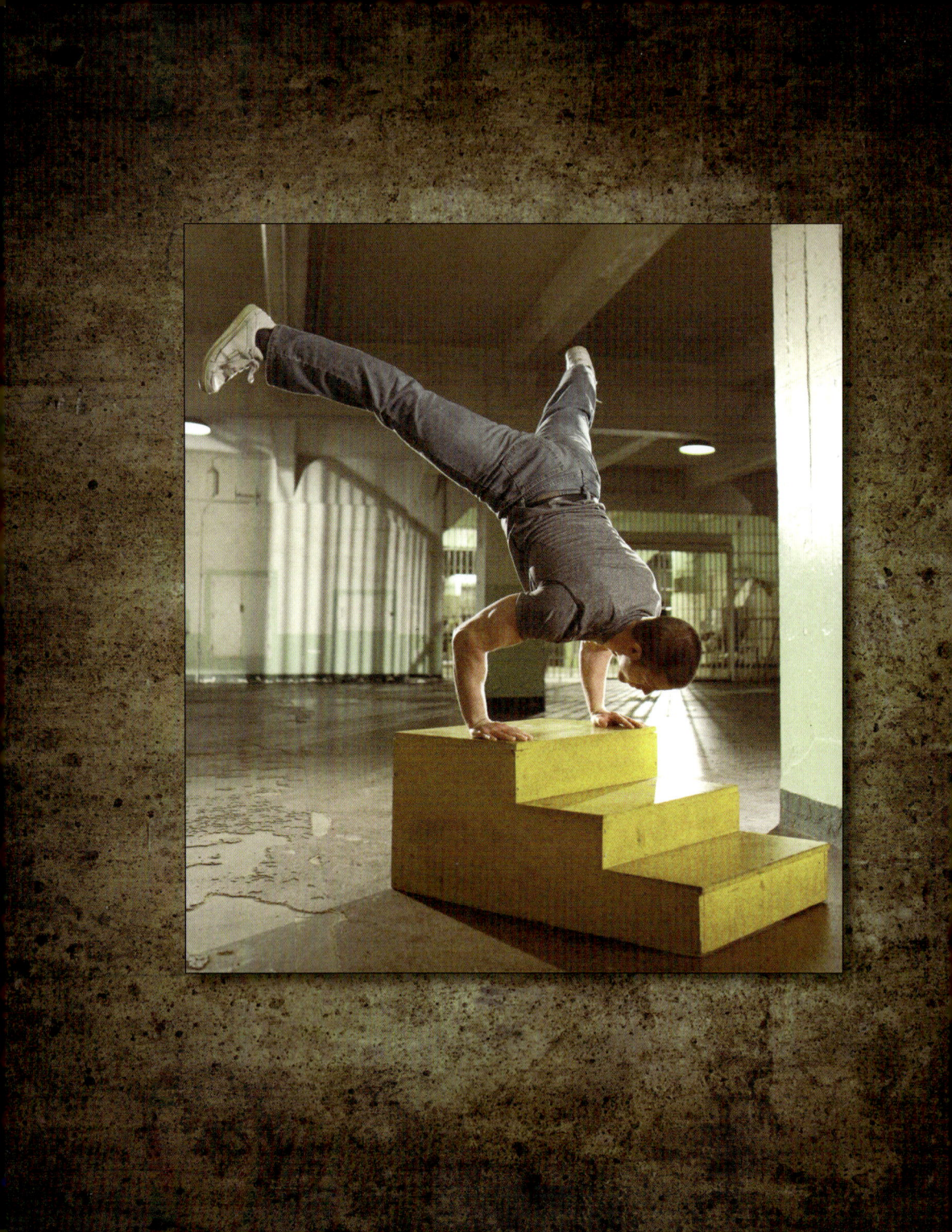

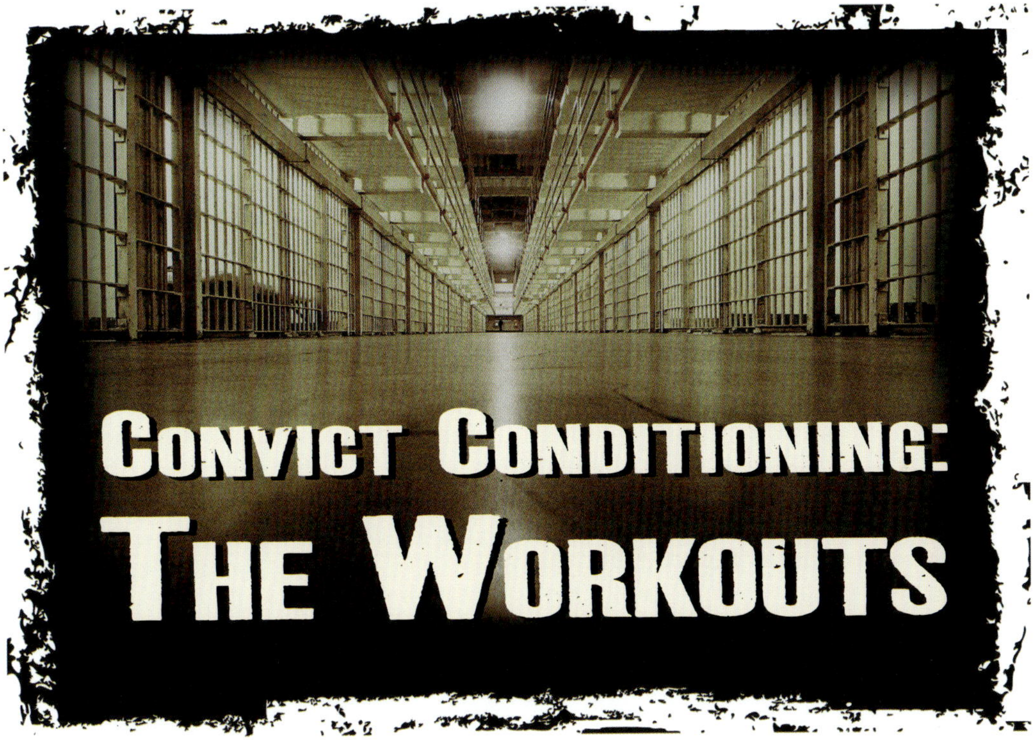

Convict Conditioning: The Workouts

In this section I'll detail six classic Convict Conditioning workout programs to get you training. No matter what level you're currently at, you'll find a program here that fits your needs.

Some people get real excited about finding the "perfect" program. I'm sad to disappoint folks who think this way, but *there is no perfect program*. Focusing too much on what program you are doing is always a mistake. To offset this tendency, I always drill the following mantra into my students: *progress, not program*.

PROGRESS, NOT PROGRAM!

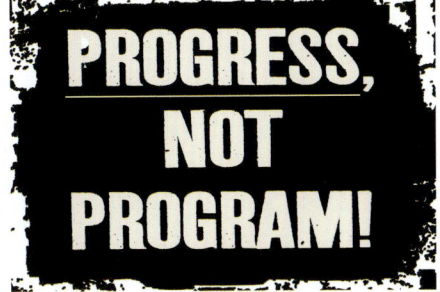

All athletes should pay attention first and foremost, not to finding the latest and "best" program, but as to whether or not they are progressing on their exercises. *Are you adding reps consistently? Is your form improving?* If so, then you are doing something right. It doesn't matter whether you are on the latest super-duper, cutting-edge, computerized championship program—if you aren't making progress, what's the point? This is the true beauty of keeping a log—it keeps you centered on your weekly *progress*, rather than focusing on whatever program you are doing at the time. A lot of athletes ask me whether they should try this or that new program, whether or not this or that workout will be overtraining or not. I always answer them the same way: try it. The only ultimate answer as to whether a program works *for you* lies in your own progress (or lack of it). Think about your progress first, and your program will eventually take care of itself.

Remember too that over time your body and your needs will change, and so will your program. For variety's sake, it's good to shake up your program every few weeks, and overhaul things every few months. Please don't think you are meant to be chained to the routines in this book—Convict Conditioning is an *approach*, not a program (or set of programs) and this approach can fit any number of different workout types and styles. Over time, as you get to learn your body, you will probably begin to make up your own programs and workouts. That's great too!

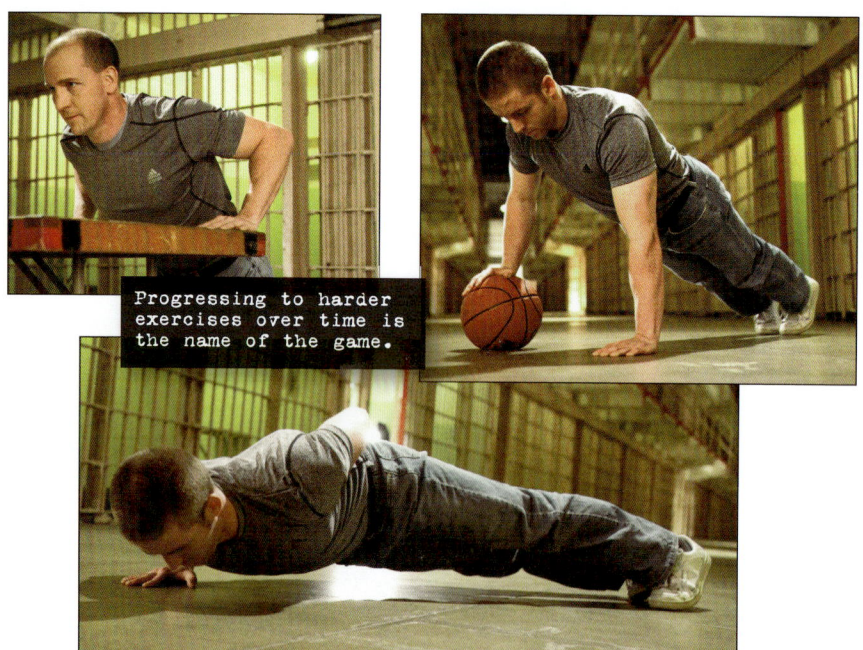

Progressing to harder exercises over time is the name of the game.

NEW BLOOD

New Blood is a great routine for beginners, or athletes who are totally new to calisthenics.

The program is condensed and abbreviated for maximum efficiency. During the week you perform just *four* basic exercises which work the whole body: *pushups* (upper-body pushing), *pullups* (upper-body pulling), *bodyweight squats* (legs and spine) and *leg raises* (midsection and hips). After warming up, perform 2-3 hard ("work") sets of each exercise, adding reps and moving to harder variations over time.

This routine allows for lots of recovery. It gives new or beaten up athletes a chance to reconnect with bodyweight movement, while safely building joint strength and muscular conditioning.

New Blood 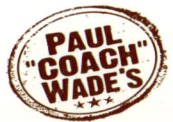 ULTIMATE BODYWEIGHT TRAINING LOG

MONDAY:	Pushups	2-3 work sets
	Leg raises	2-3 work sets
TUESDAY:	Off	
WEDNESDAY:	Off	
THURSDAY:	Off	
FRIDAY:	Pullups	2-3 work sets
	Squats	2-3 work sets
SATURDAY:	Off	
SUNDAY:	Off	

GOOD BEHAVIOR

Good Behavior is an ideal routine for any athlete beyond the intermediate stage who wishes to gain strength and muscle.

Good Behavior builds on the *New Blood* program. You still work each exercise once per week for maximum recovery and muscle growth, but now you add two more advanced exercises into the mix: *handstand pushups* (for shoulder strength/pressing power) and *bridges* (spinal flexibility and posterior chain strength). As with all these programs, warm up well with a set or two of lighter exercises before hitting 2 "work" sets of each exercise.

There is very little training overlap on this routine, and plenty of rest, making it an excellent strength program for athletes who train in other sports (MMA, wrestling, climbing, boxing, etc).

GOOD BEHAVIOR 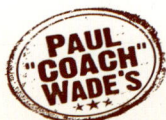 ULTIMATE BODYWEIGHT TRAINING LOG

MONDAY:	Pushups	2 work sets
	Leg raises	2 work sets
TUESDAY:	Off	
WEDNESDAY:	Pullups	2 work sets
	Squats	2 work sets
THURSDAY:	Off	
FRIDAY:	Handstand pushups	2 work sets
	Bridges	2 work sets
SATURDAY:	Off	
SUNDAY:	Off	

VETERANO

Veterano is an unconventional program that any intermediate athlete can experiment with.

On the *Veterano* routine you work the six major movements of strength calisthenics, focusing only on one each day. For maximum recovery, you should alternate upper and lower-body exercises wherever possible: you do squats on one day, pushups the next, and so on. The *Veterano* template can take a lot of tweaking; you can add extra sets, extra variant exercises, extra rest days as and when you like, without screwing up the basic structure.

Because you are working just one movement each day, this routine is a real life-saver for athletes who complain that they don't have time to train. Each workout can take as little as six or seven minutes!

Veterano

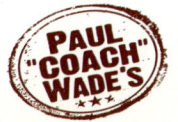

ULTIMATE BODYWEIGHT TRAINING LOG

MONDAY:	Pullups	2-3 work sets
TUESDAY:	Bridges	2-3 work sets
WEDNESDAY:	Handstand pushups	2-3 work sets
THURSDAY:	Leg raises	2-3 work sets
FRIDAY:	Squats	2-3 work sets
SATURDAY:	Pushups	2-3 work sets
SUNDAY:	Off	

HARD TIME

Hard Time is a very balanced strength and muscle-building program which can work well for intermediate and advanced athletes.

In *Hard Time* you work two upper-body pushing movements per week (*pushups, handstand pushups*) and two upper-body pulling movements (*pullups, horizontal pulls*). In between this session you hit the lower body hard with *bridges, leg raises* and *squats*.

This program is pretty upper-body heavy, and will prove effective for somebody in a hurry to add lots of strength and beef to the torso and arms. Because the lower body only gets one session each week, the routine also works very well for athletes who already work their lower body a lot: runners, cyclists, karate practitioners, etc.

Hard Time 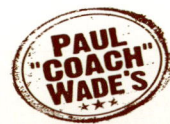 ULTIMATE BODYWEIGHT TRAINING LOG

MONDAY:	Pullups	2-3 work sets
	Handstand pushups	2-3 work sets
TUESDAY:	Off	
WEDNESDAY:	Bridges	2-3 work sets
	Leg raises	2-3 work sets
	Squats	2-3 work sets
THURSDAY:	Off	
FRIDAY:	Pushups	2-3 work sets
	Horizontal pulls	2-3 work sets
SATURDAY:		Off

REVOLVING DOOR

Recovery and recuperation are crucial factors in all strength training—you grow when you *rest*, not when you *train*. But some experienced athletes have the drive and the recovery ability to work the body more frequently than most mortals. This is where the *Revolving Door* program comes in.

On this program you work on the "Big Six" calisthenics exercises: *pushups, squats, pullups, leg raises, bridges* and *handstand pushups*. You perform three of these movements per session, taking a day off after each workout. This means you wind up doing either three or four workouts per week. Since some of these exercises overlap (e.g., *pushups* and *handstand pushups*) you will actually be working some muscles *four times* or more over an eight day period.

This is too much for most people, but if you have the recovery ability to handle the increased workload, this routine will take you to the elite level—fast.

Revolving Door 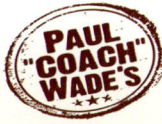 ULTIMATE BODYWEIGHT TRAINING LOG

DAY 1:	Pullups	2-3 work sets
	Squats	2-3 work sets
	Pushups	2-3 work sets
DAY 2:	Off	
DAY 3:	Handstand pushups	2-3 work sets
	Bridges	2-3 work sets
	Leg raises	2-3 work sets
Day 4:	Off	

Continue to revolve the two workouts with a day off in between

LOCKDOWN

As the name suggests, this program is only for those calisthenics experts who have got their training totally locked down. Advanced athletes only need apply!

You train four days per week. On two of those days you perform upper-body and waist work. On the remaining two days you work the lower body, blasting your wheels with *one-leg squats*, and finishing them off with either explosive work (*box jumps, tuck jumps, dead leaps, one-leg jumps, vaulting*, etc.), or endurance training (*runs, sprints, hill sprints, car pushing*, etc). Advanced athletes should begin supplementing *front levers* for *horizontal pulls*.

Lockdown is my personal favorite Convict Conditioning program. It's definitely not for everyone, but the athlete who can stay the course will win it all—strength, muscle, stamina, agility and power. Total bodyweight mastery.

Lockdown 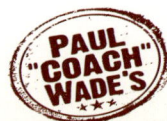 Ultimate Bodyweight Training Log

MONDAY:	Pullups	2-3 work sets
	Handstand pushups	2-3 work sets
	Leg raises/twists	various
TUESDAY:	One-leg squats	5 work sets
	Explosive leg work	up to 10 sets
WEDNESDAY:	Off	
THURSDAY:	Pushups	2-3 work sets
	Horizontal pulls	2-3 work sets
	Bridges/twists	various
FRIDAY:	One-leg squats	5 work sets
	Endurance leg work	various
SATURDAY:		Off
SUNDAY:		Off

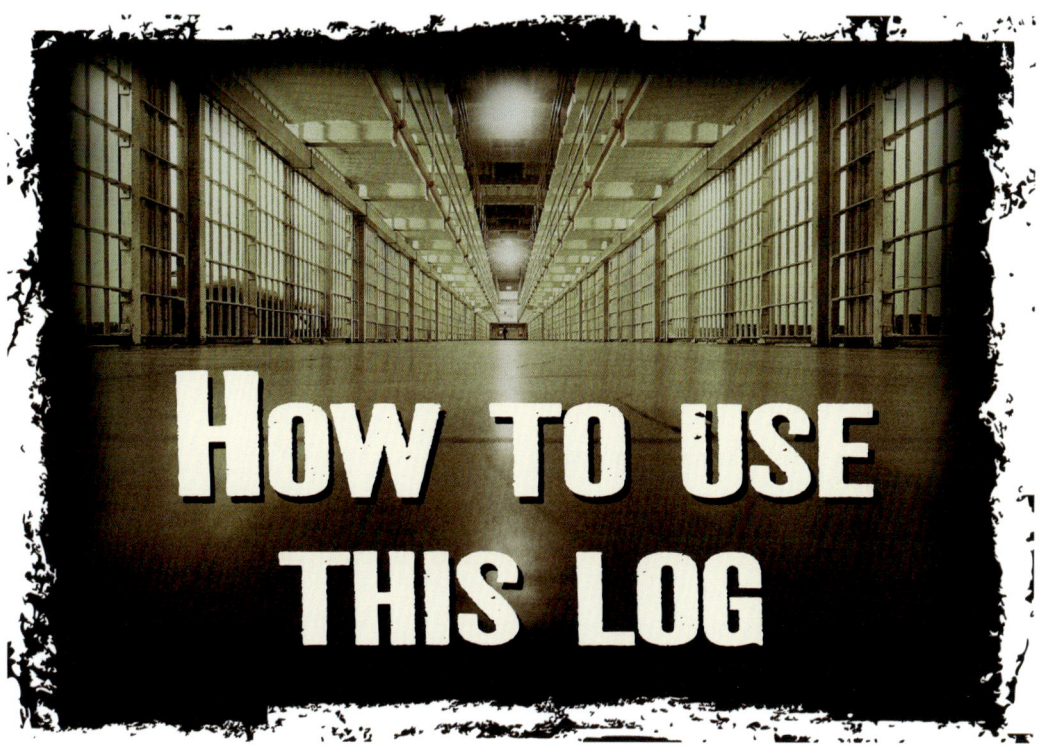

How to Use This Log

This log is designed after the kind of bodyweight journal a lot of convict-athletes construct for themselves. This means that there's no bull—no calorie counters, no blood pressure stats, no supplements list. A log should be just the facts, with as little fancy crap as possible to distract you from the real thing: *brutally hard bodyweight training*. This is exactly what this log is all about.

This log is also designed to be as flexible as you want. A lot of journals are built like *diaries*, with seven daily one-page entries making up a week. This inevitably amounts to a huge waste of space, since strength athletes need more recovery time than many other sportspeople. Hard-working strength athletes (even many pros) train on average three days per week, meaning that trainees are forced to leave four out of every seven pages empty. By the time you have done with some of these logs, they are more than half blank! In this log, you fill in one entry per workout, leaving no wasted space.

Actually completing an entry couldn't be simpler. After a workout, you write down:

    A. The day/date

    B. The exercises you performed

    C. The reps you did for each set

    D. Any extra training or work you did (not compulsory)

    E. Any notes/comments you want to record (not compulsory)

With a log like this example on the next page there are zero excuses—recording your workouts could not be any easier.

Get doing those pushups, kid.

ULTIMATE TRAINING LOG

21

DAY: Thursday
DATE: 3/7/2013

NO.	EXERCISE	SET 1	SET 2	SET 3	SET 4	SET 5
1	Incline Pushups (warmup)	20				
2	Full Pushups (warm up)	15				
3	Uneven Pushups	18	16			
4	Supported Squats (warm up)	20	26			
5	Close Squats (warm up)	12				
6	Assisted one-leg Squats	16	11			
7	Wall Squat	60's				
8	Jackknife Pullups (warm up)	15				
9	Uneven Pullups (left)	7	6			
	Uneven Pullups (right)	7	5			
10	Burpees (with jump)	5	10	15	20	15
		10	5			
11	Deep Breathing	10	12			

EXTRAS:
Did the Trifecta several times through the day

COMMENTS:
Did an extra warm up on the squats. Lower back feeling better; need to improve form on the pushups.

Annotations:
- A. Insert the Day and Date
- B. List the exercises you worked with
- C. Record how many reps you did for Set 1, Set 2, Set 3, etc.
- If you perform holds, you can fill in TIME instead of reps
- If you run out of room, just start again on the next line (or next page).
- D. Write down any extra training or workload.
- E. Put any comments here.

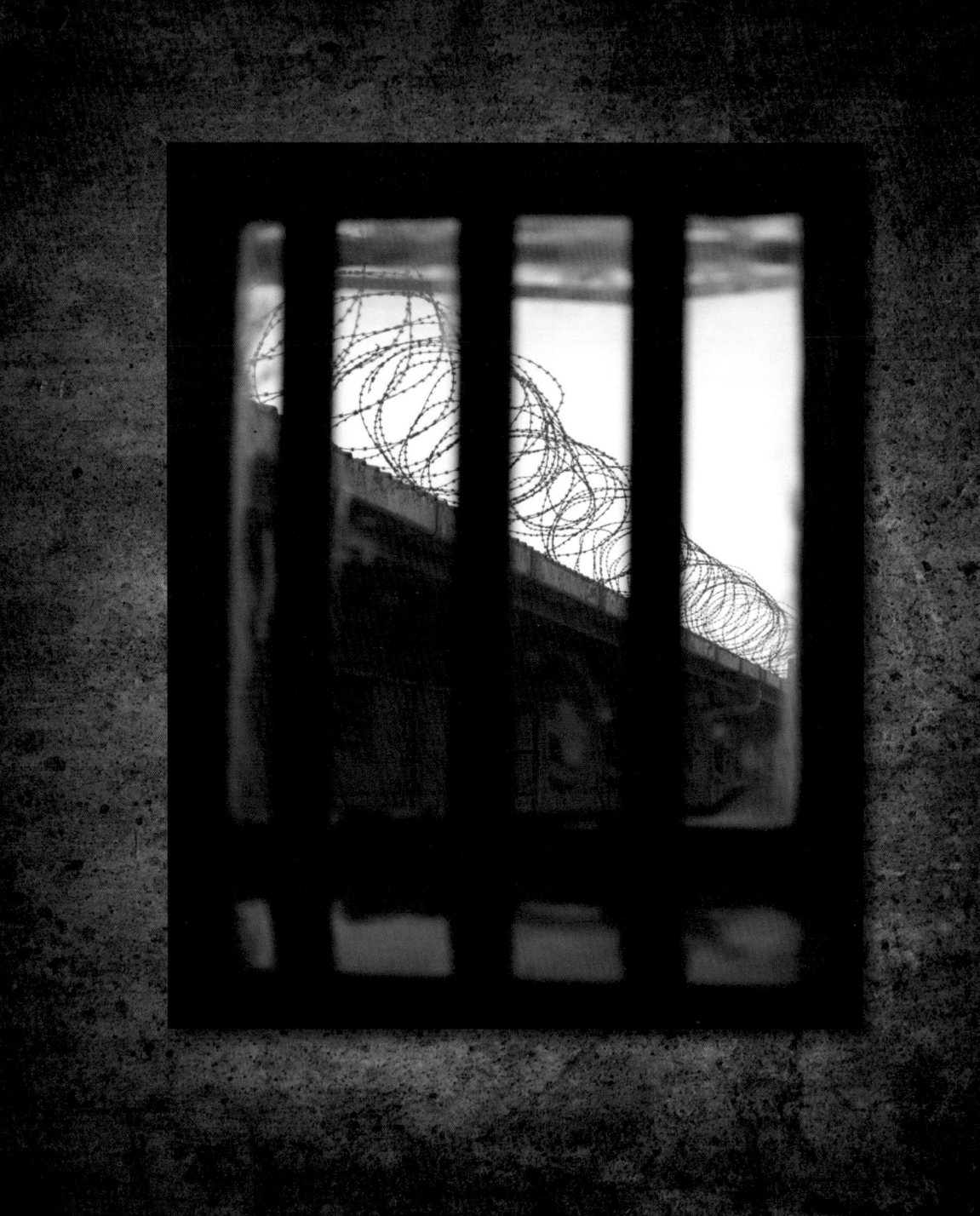

Part II:
Log Entries

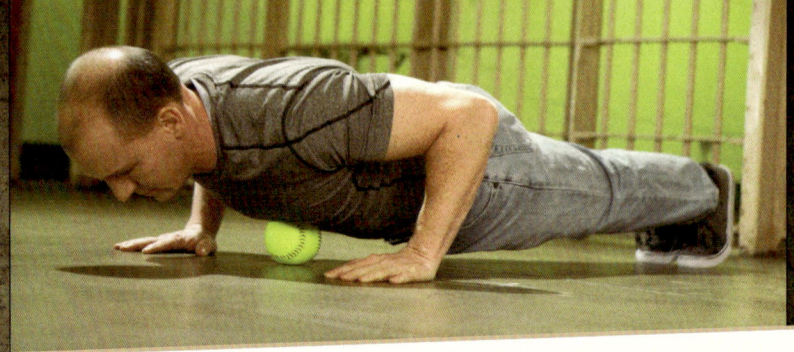

ON WORKOUT LENGTH:

When you fill out a workout log entry, don't worry about filling out the entire page. A workout should be measured by its *intensity* and *quality*, not by how many exercises you perform! A single set of a hundred pushups makes for a helluva workout…although it doesn't even fill one line of a log page, how many athletes could handle a workout with that kind of brutal intensity?

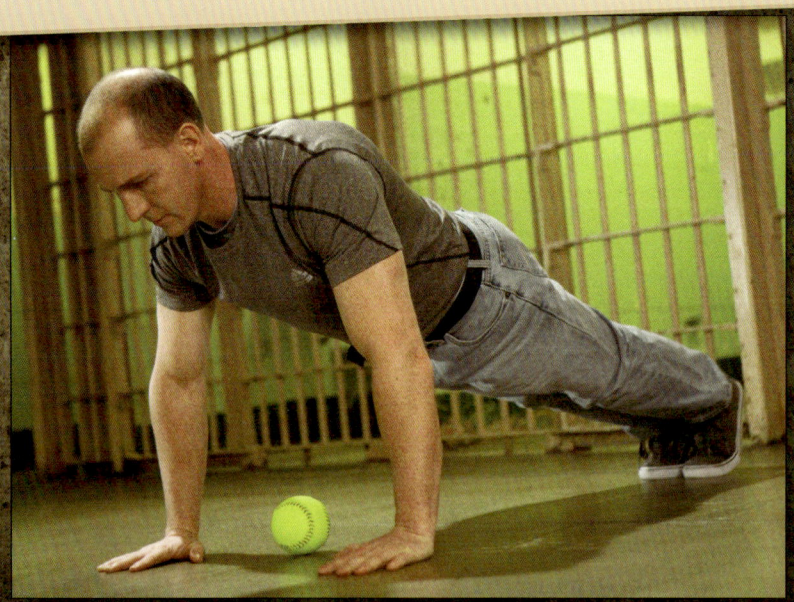

CONVICT CONDITIONING — Ultimate Bodyweight TRAINING LOG

DAY: _____

DATE: _____

NO.	EXERCISE	SET 1	SET 2	SET 3	SET 4	SET 5

EXTRAS:

COMMENTS:

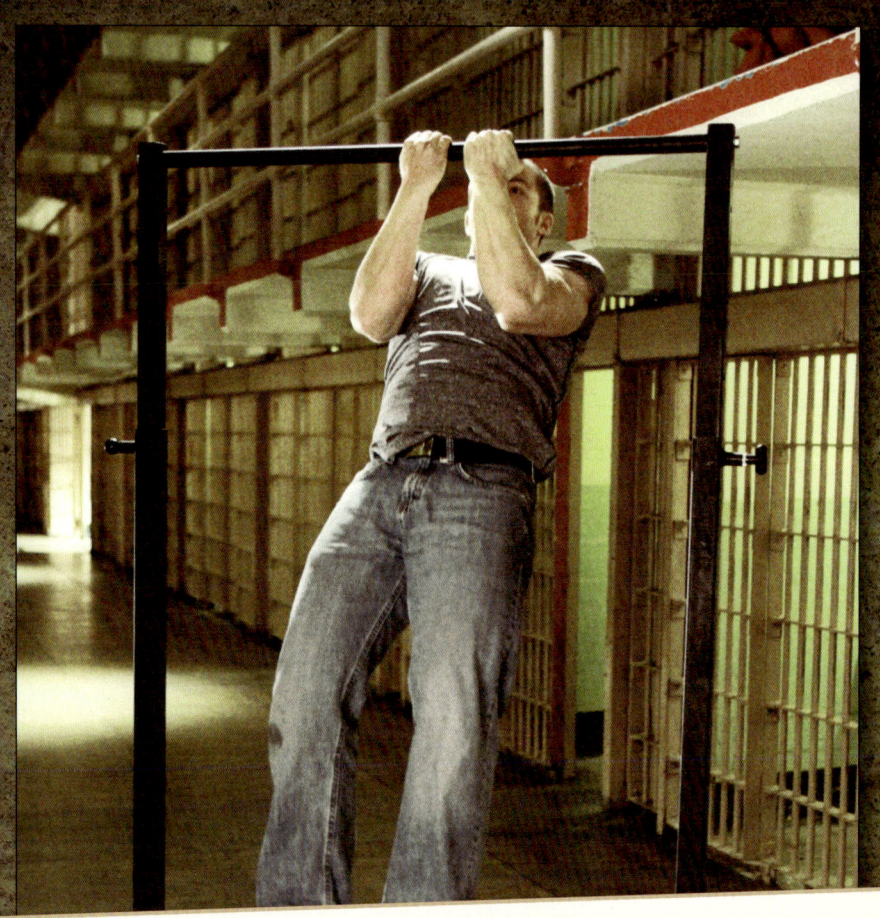

ON STRONG BICEPS:

Most athletes head straight for barbell curls in an attempt to build strong biceps. Curls are usually labeled as a "compound" movement, but in reality they are an *isolation* movement—they force the biceps to work in an anatomically weak position. The biceps evolved to work in a pullup-type motion, and this is where they are strongest. Very few men can curl 200 lbs, but most healthy 200 lbs males can do a pullup. For true biceps power, head to the overhead bar!

CONVICT CONDITIONING — Ultimate Bodyweight Training Log

DAY: _____
DATE: _____

27

NO.	EXERCISE	SET 1	SET 2	SET 3	SET 4	SET 5

EXTRAS:

COMMENTS:

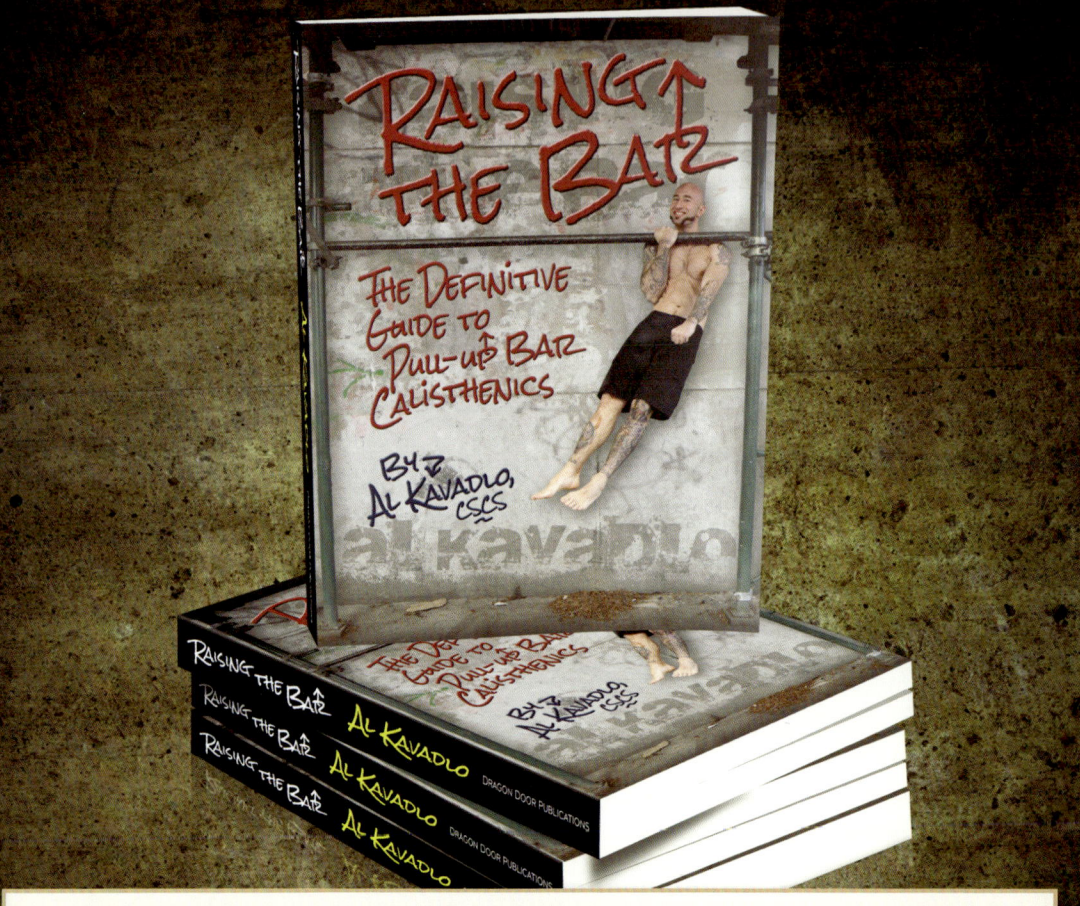

Great Bodyweight Strength Books # 1:
Raising the Bar—Al Kavadlo

Al Kavadlo is rapidly becoming an icon in the calisthenics world. An incredible athlete, Al is also a genius coach and innovator who can *talk the talk* as well as *walk the walk*. In 2012 Al wrote *Raising the Bar,* the first ever manual of bar calisthenics, and the most important fitness publishing event in decades. The book quickly became a must-have, not only because of its unique information, but because of the feedback coming from users. Al Kavadlo and his brother Danny represent the future of bodyweight training, and fitness in general. Buy this book!

CONVICT CONDITIONING
Ultimate Bodyweight Training Log

DAY: _____
DATE: _____

NO.	EXERCISE	SET 1	SET 2	SET 3	SET 4	SET 5

EXTRAS:

COMMENTS:

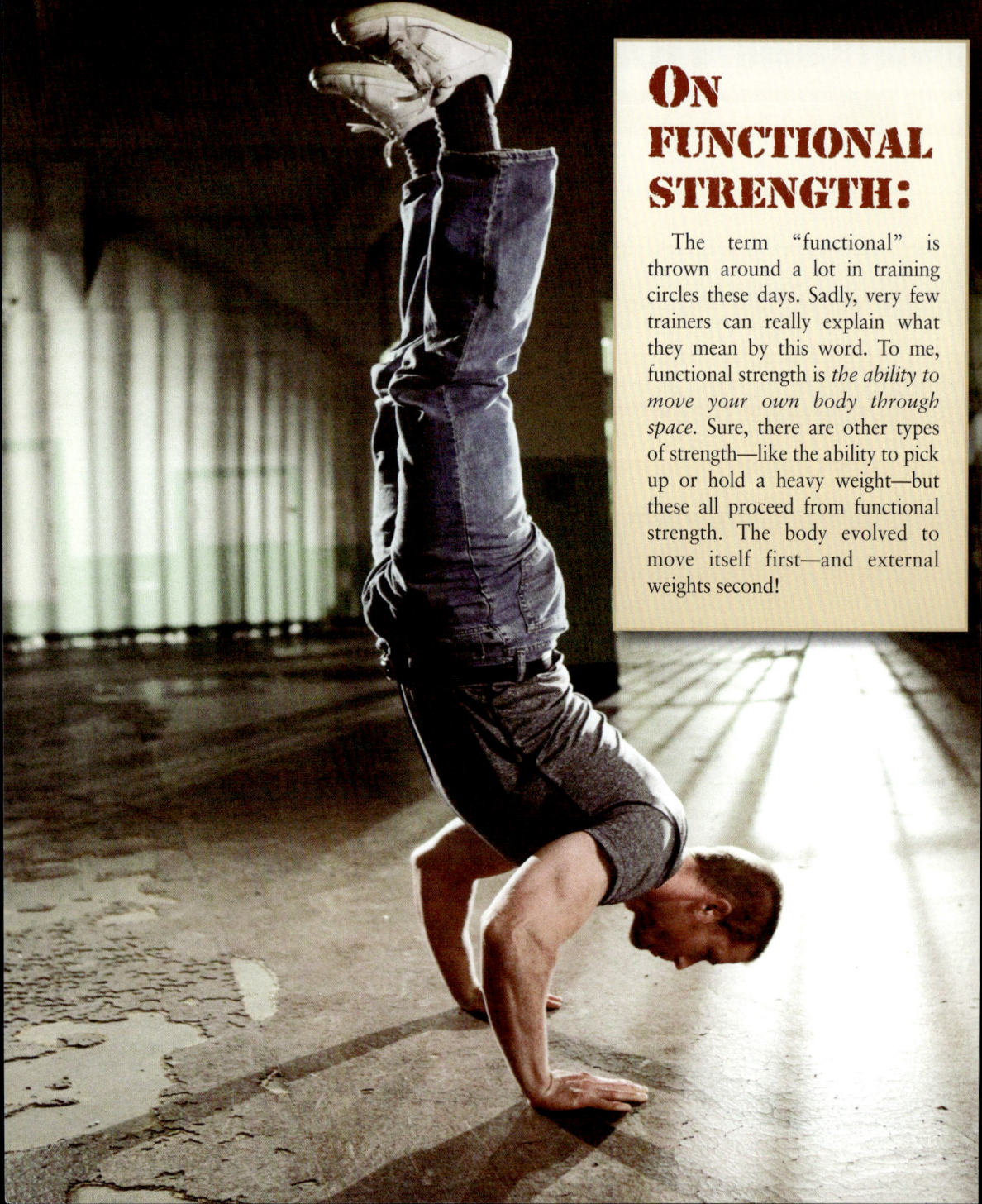

ON FUNCTIONAL STRENGTH:

The term "functional" is thrown around a lot in training circles these days. Sadly, very few trainers can really explain what they mean by this word. To me, functional strength is *the ability to move your own body through space*. Sure, there are other types of strength—like the ability to pick up or hold a heavy weight—but these all proceed from functional strength. The body evolved to move itself first—and external weights second!

CONVICT CONDITIONING — Ultimate Bodyweight Training Log

31

DAY: _____
DATE: _____

NO.	EXERCISE	SET 1	SET 2	SET 3	SET 4	SET 5

EXTRAS:

COMMENTS:

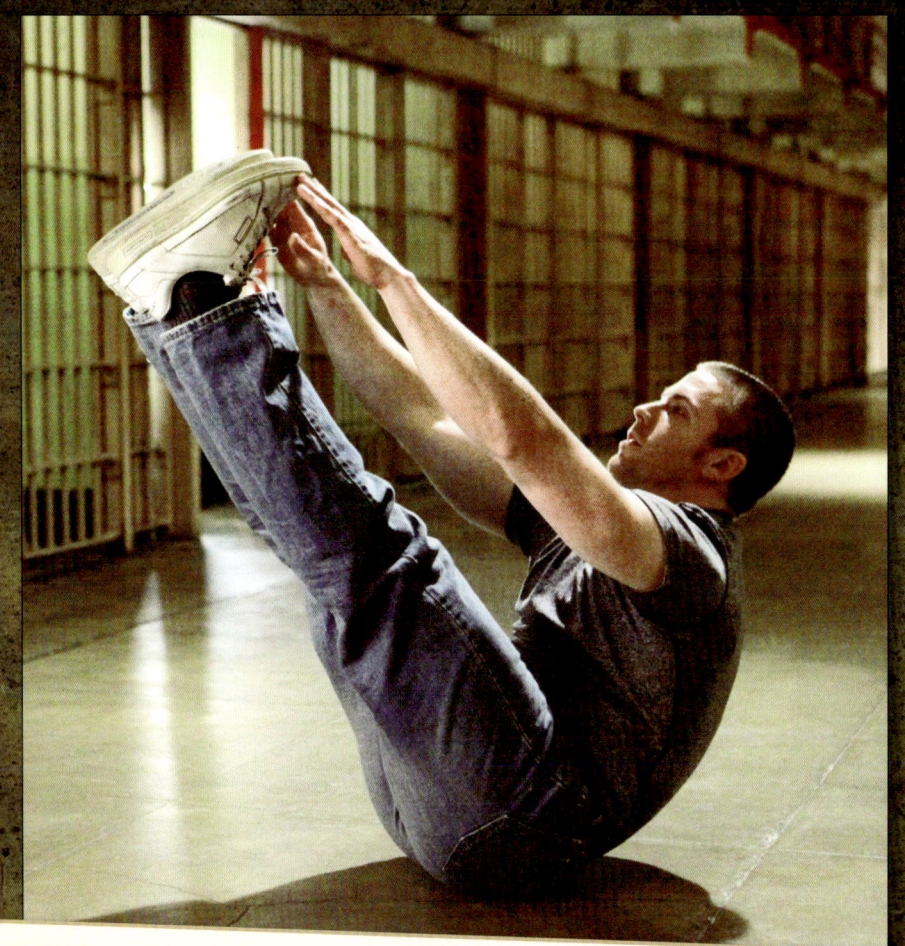

ON TIGHT ABS:

All the old-time strongmen used to pull their *guts in tight* during midsection training or "gut work". Doing this trains the internal abdominal muscles (the *transversus*). Modern bodybuilders are only concerned with working the superficial layer of muscle (the *rectus abdominis*), and as a result they often have hanging bellies, no matter how lean and "ripped" their stomach appears. Consciously suck your gut in when you train abs, from the first rep to the last!

PAUL "COACH" WADE'S CONVICT CONDITIONING
Ultimate Bodyweight Training Log

33

DAY: _____
DATE: _____

NO.	EXERCISE	SET 1	SET 2	SET 3	SET 4	SET 5

EXTRAS:

COMMENTS:

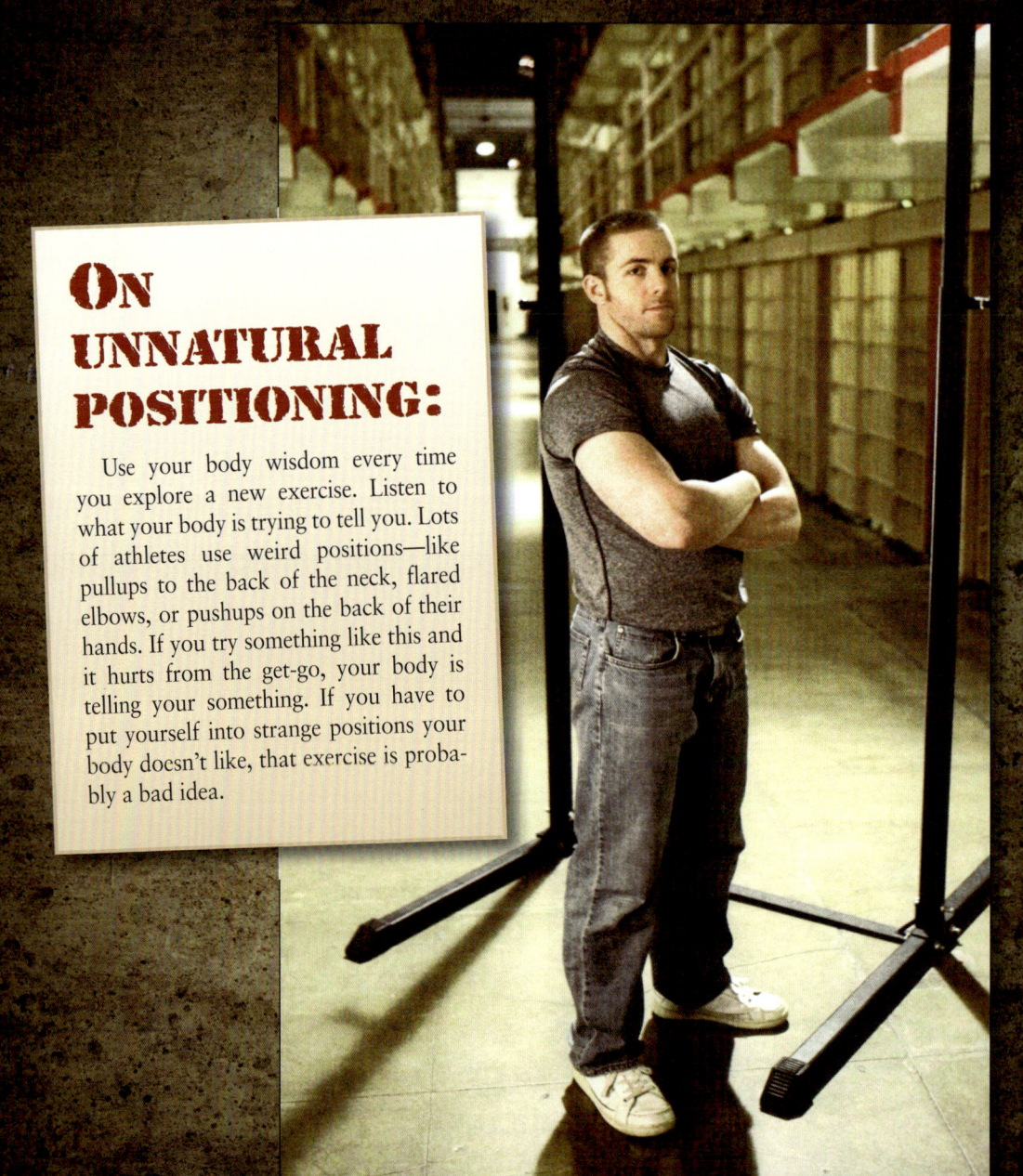

ON UNNATURAL POSITIONING:

Use your body wisdom every time you explore a new exercise. Listen to what your body is trying to tell you. Lots of athletes use weird positions—like pullups to the back of the neck, flared elbows, or pushups on the back of their hands. If you try something like this and it hurts from the get-go, your body is telling your something. If you have to put yourself into strange positions your body doesn't like, that exercise is probably a bad idea.

PAUL "COACH" WADE'S CONVICT CONDITIONING — Ultimate Bodyweight Training Log

DAY: _____

DATE: _____

NO.	EXERCISE	SET 1	SET 2	SET 3	SET 4	SET 5

EXTRAS:

COMMENTS:

ON PARTNER WORK:

Partner calisthenics--so loved by the old-time strongmen--is sadly neglected by isolated modern trainees. With a partner you can do flags, handstands, carries and midsection work; hundreds of techniques exist for creative minds. Back in the day, even convicts got into the act; in San Quentin in the 40s, there was a regular calisthenics team who met in the yard to train together. Their abilities became so impressive they were even featured in *Strength & Health* magazine.

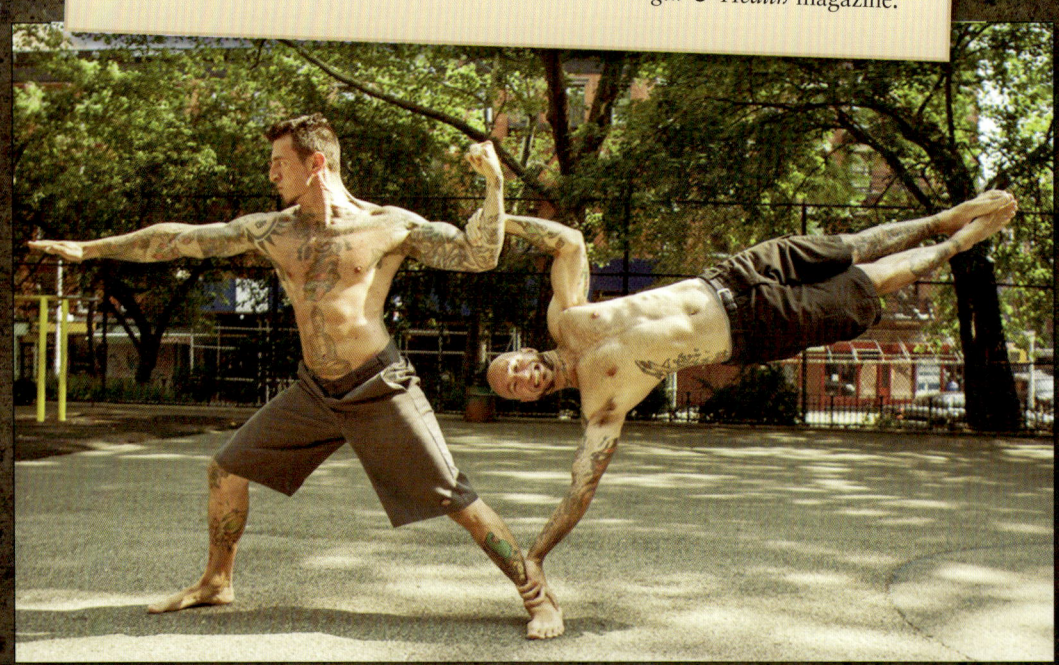

CONVICT CONDITIONING — Ultimate Bodyweight Training Log

PAUL "COACH" WADE'S

DAY: _____

DATE: _____

NO.	EXERCISE	SET 1	SET 2	SET 3	SET 4	SET 5

EXTRAS:

COMMENTS:

On Wall Squats:

Wall squats—known by the old-time strongmen as "Samson's Seat"—are a great example of static strength work for the lower body. Just lean back against a wall with your thighs parallel to the ground and hold the position as long as possible, breathing smoothly. As your strength and endurance build, you can go deeper, and ultimately try the exercise on one leg. Makes for a great finisher.

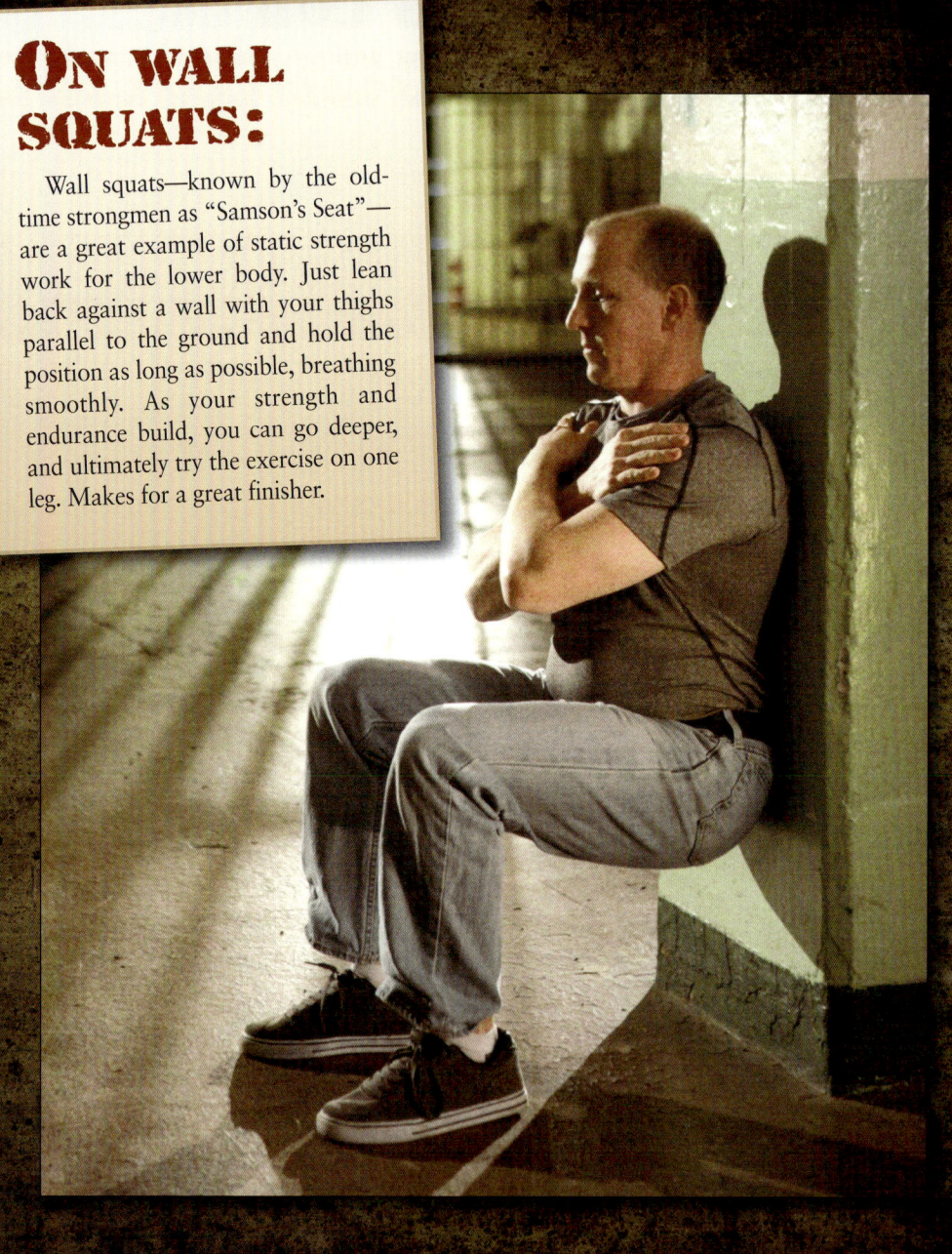

PAUL "COACH" WADE'S CONVICT CONDITIONING ULTIMATE BODYWEIGHT TRAINING LOG

DAY: _____

DATE: _____

NO.	EXERCISE	SET 1	SET 2	SET 3	SET 4	SET 5

EXTRAS:

COMMENTS:

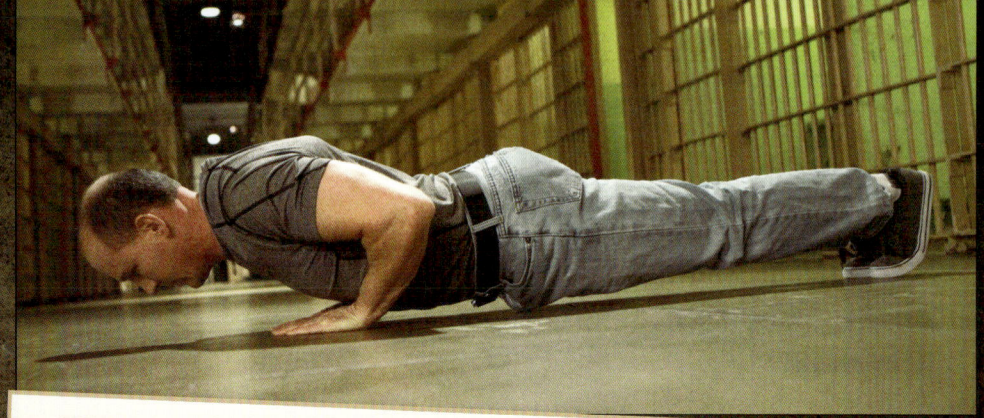

ON HAND PLACEMENT:

As a general rule, the deltoid muscles work optimally when the hands are *wide*, the torso muscles work optimally when the hands are *shoulder-width*, and the arm muscles work optimally when the hands are *close together*. Since the torso muscles (chest, lats and back) are the strongest upper-body muscles, most athletes are at their strongest with a grip or hand placement that is approximately shoulder-width during training.

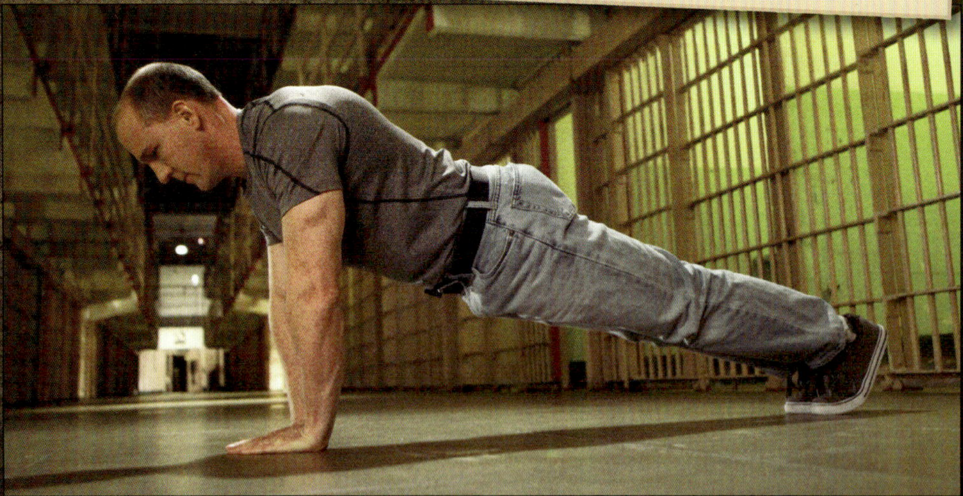

CONVICT CONDITIONING
Ultimate Bodyweight Training Log

DAY: _____
DATE: _____

NO.	EXERCISE	SET 1	SET 2	SET 3	SET 4	SET 5

EXTRAS:

COMMENTS:

ON BOUNCING:

Unless you are exploring explosive training methods, don't ever bounce during the bottom of a calisthenics movement. If you are bouncing, you are using momentum, and if momentum is doing the work *your muscles aren't*. Bouncing not only harms your progress, on exercises like squats it can seriously damage the joints. Countless knee cartilage tears have occurred due to bouncing out of deep squats.

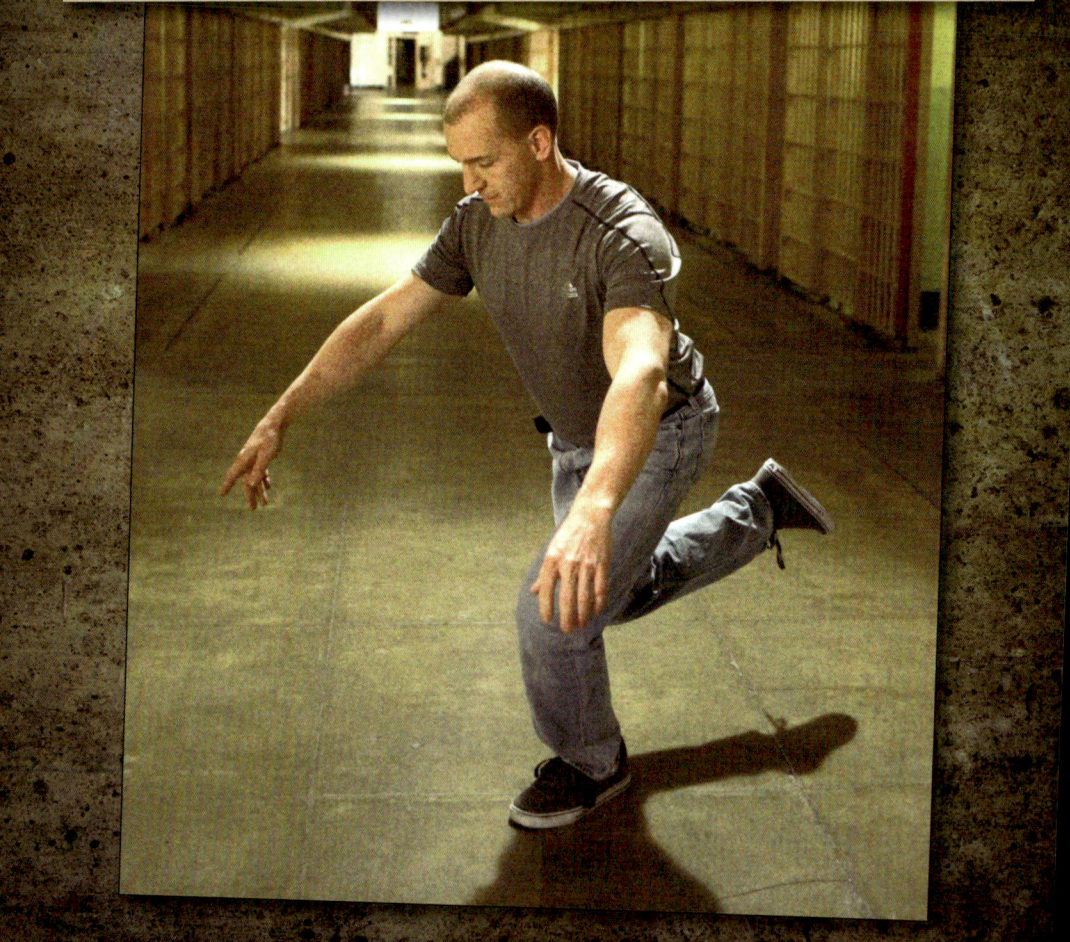

PAUL "COACH" WADE'S CONVICT CONDITIONING
Ultimate Bodyweight Training Log

DAY: _____

DATE: _____

NO.	EXERCISE	SET 1	SET 2	SET 3	SET 4	SET 5

EXTRAS:

COMMENTS:

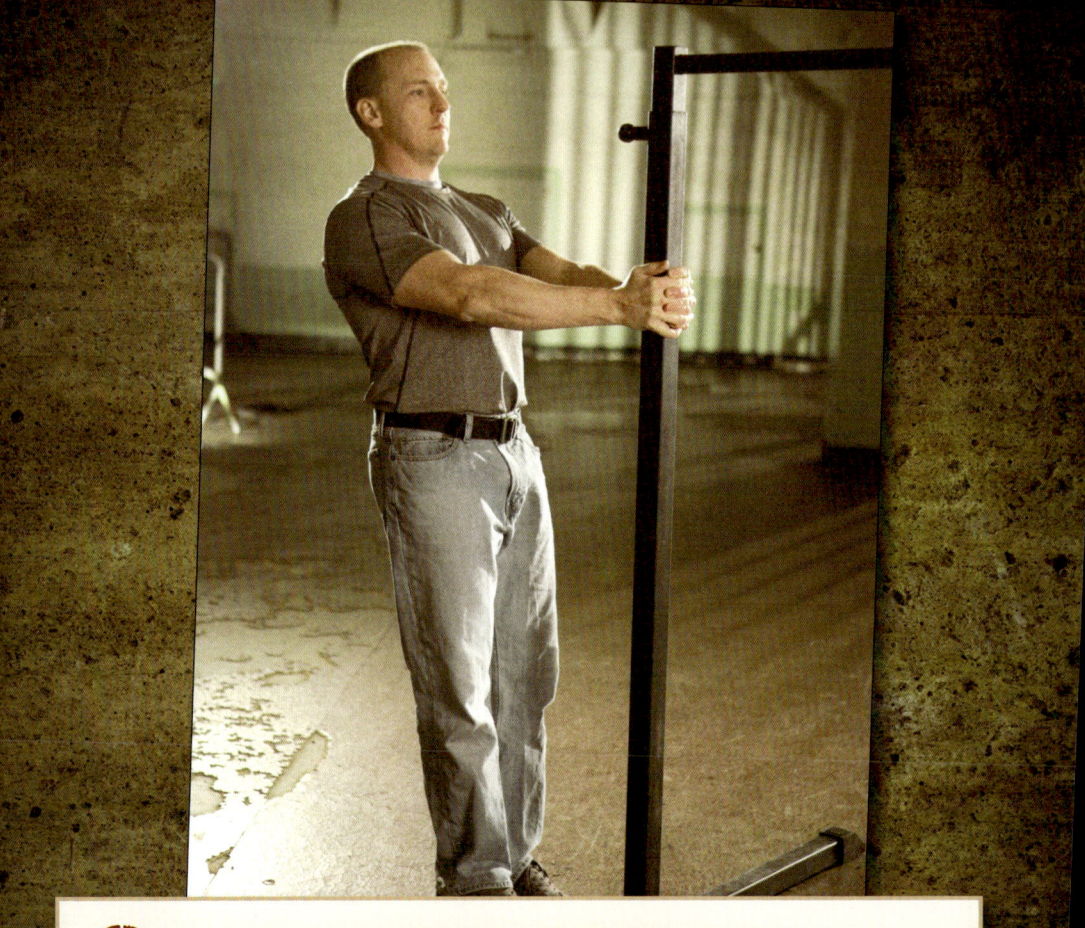

On starting easy:

If you want to really build maximum levels of strength, you should always start your training with the easiest exercises, and improve gradually. This method not only builds the joints, and teaches good form, it also banks strength and generates a huge amount of momentum. Many powerlifting systems also advise beginning the program from a very easy base for optimal gains in the long run. Jim Wendler's popular 5/3/1 system is one such example.

PAUL "COACH" WADE'S CONVICT CONDITIONING
Ultimate Bodyweight Training Log

DAY: _____
DATE: _____

45

NO.	EXERCISE	SET 1	SET 2	SET 3	SET 4	SET 5

EXTRAS:

COMMENTS:

ON SHOULDERS:

The shoulders have evolved to work as an incredibly mobile, versatile joint; unfortunately, most athletes only use them to push and pull in straight lines. No wonder the shoulders stiffen up on strong folks. To keep the deep tissues of your shoulders healthy and mobile, include circular and twisting movements in your workouts. You don't need rubber bands or similar gadgets—just move your body.

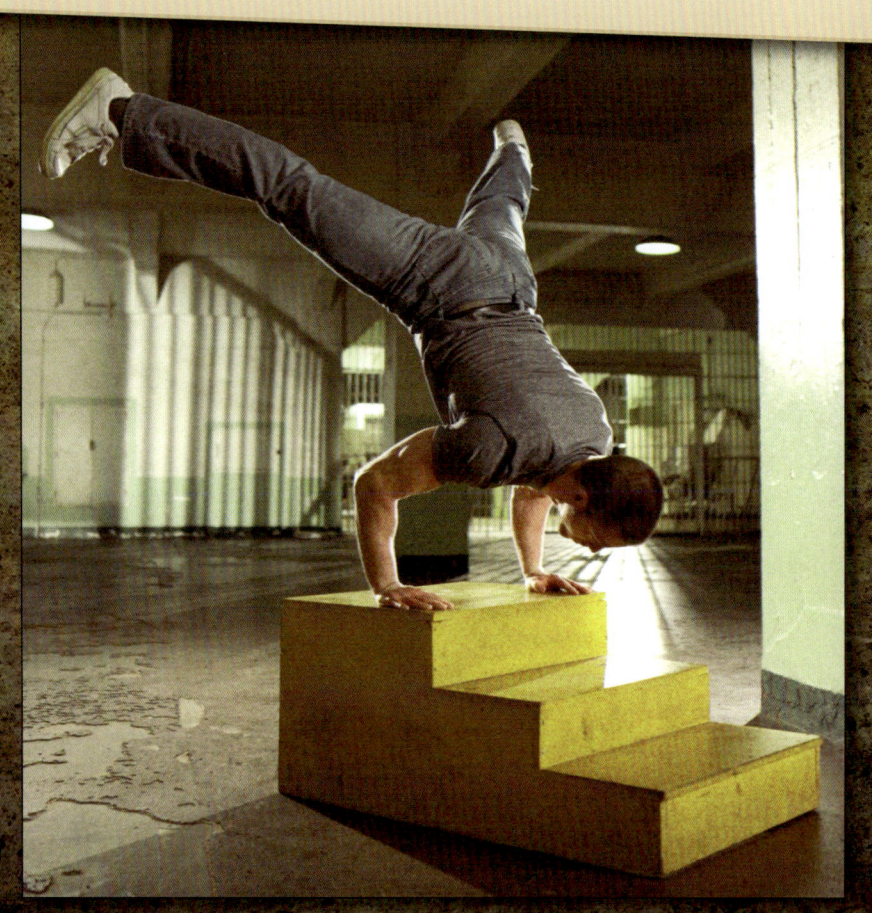

PAUL "COACH" WADE'S CONVICT CONDITIONING ULTIMATE BODYWEIGHT TRAINING LOG

DAY: _____

DATE: _____

NO.	EXERCISE	SET 1	SET 2	SET 3	SET 4	SET 5

EXTRAS:

COMMENTS:

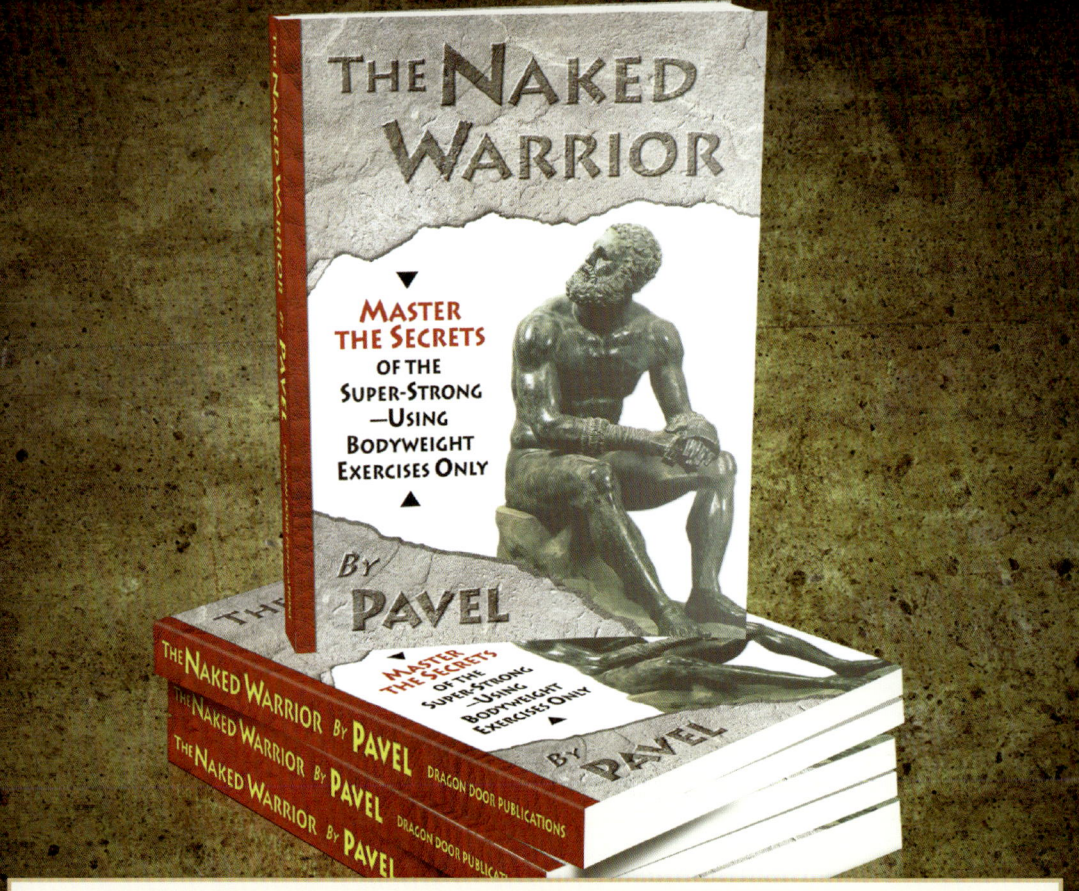

Great Bodyweight Strength Books # 2: The Naked Warrior—Pavel

In my opinion Pavel Tsatsouline is the man responsible for the current resurgence of interest in bodyweight strength training in America and Europe. Hailed by many as the world's greatest strength writer, countless athletes sat up and paid attention when he applied his methods to calisthenics in the now-classic manual *The Naked Warrior.* Challenging and brilliant, this book belongs on the shelf of every coach and athlete.

PAUL "COACH" WADE'S CONVICT CONDITIONING — Ultimate Bodyweight Training Log

DAY: _____

DATE: _____

NO.	EXERCISE	SET 1	SET 2	SET 3	SET 4	SET 5

EXTRAS:

COMMENTS:

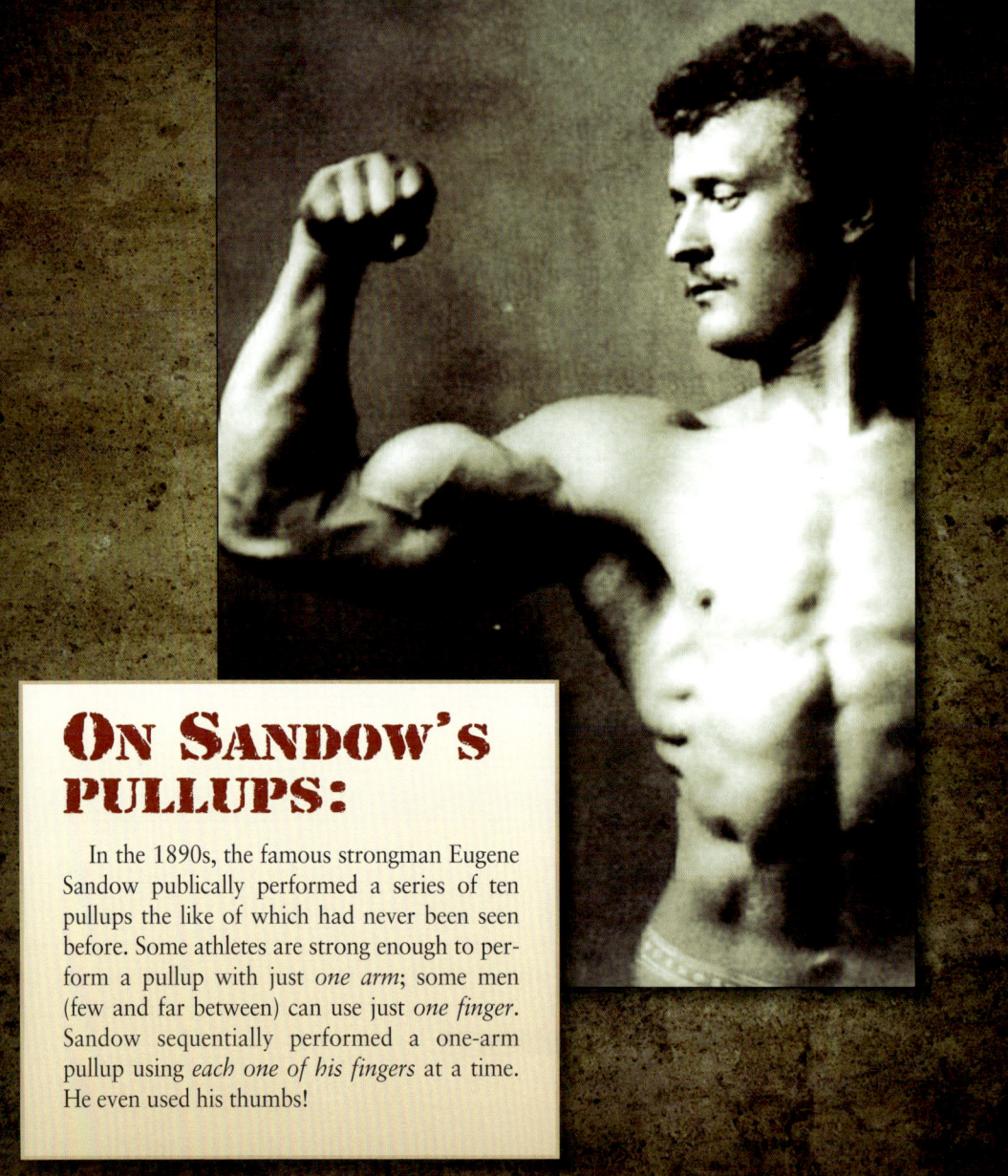

ON SANDOW'S PULLUPS:

In the 1890s, the famous strongman Eugene Sandow publically performed a series of ten pullups the like of which had never been seen before. Some athletes are strong enough to perform a pullup with just *one arm*; some men (few and far between) can use just *one finger*. Sandow sequentially performed a one-arm pullup using *each one of his fingers* at a time. He even used his thumbs!

PAUL "COACH" WADE'S CONVICT CONDITIONING
Ultimate Bodyweight Training Log

DAY: _____

DATE: _____

NO.	EXERCISE	SET 1	SET 2	SET 3	SET 4	SET 5

EXTRAS:

COMMENTS:

ON EXERCISE AND WEIGHT LOSS:

You should be training regularly for strength, mobility and health—not weight loss. A pound of fat equals around 3,500 calories; one perfect pushup burns around 0.9 calories. That means you'd need to squeeze out nearly *four thousand* pushups just to lose a single pound of fat! Don't waste your time and energy trying to lose extra fat through exercise. Instead, use nutrition: take in just 500 fewer calories than you burn each day, and you'll lose that pound of fat in a week, without much effort.

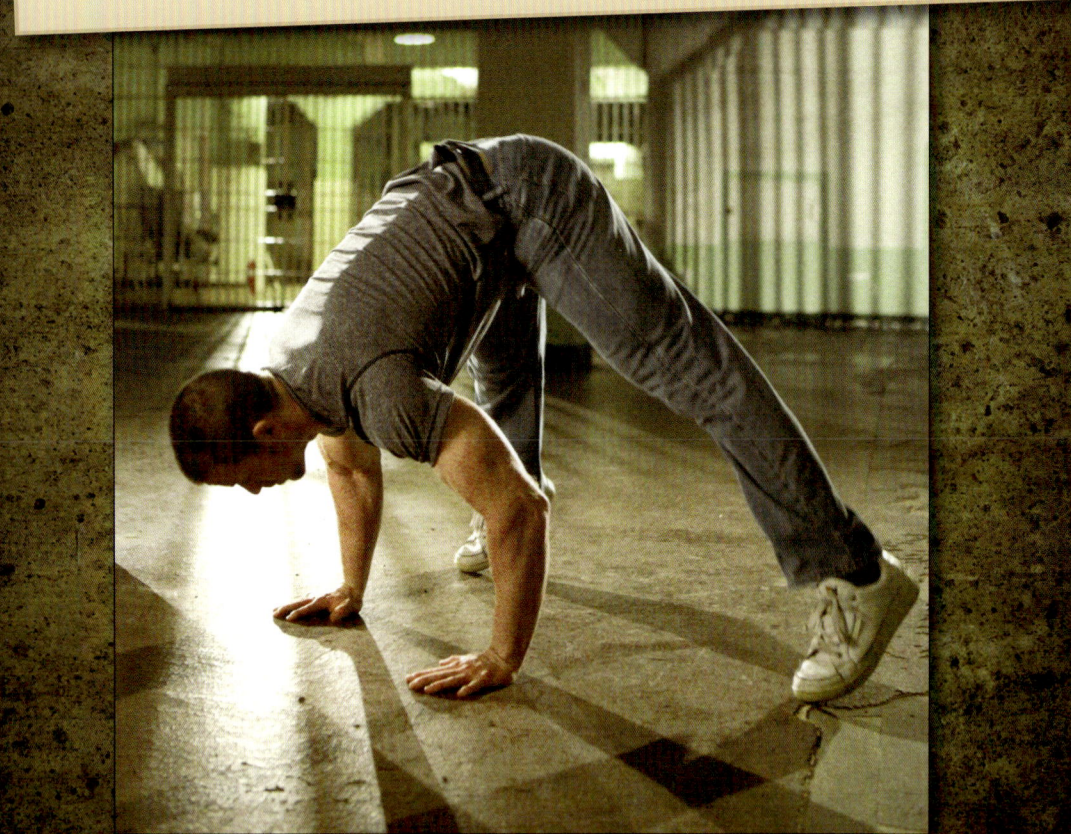

CONVICT CONDITIONING — Ultimate Bodyweight Training Log

DAY: _____
DATE: _____

NO.	EXERCISE	SET 1	SET 2	SET 3	SET 4	SET 5

EXTRAS:

COMMENTS:

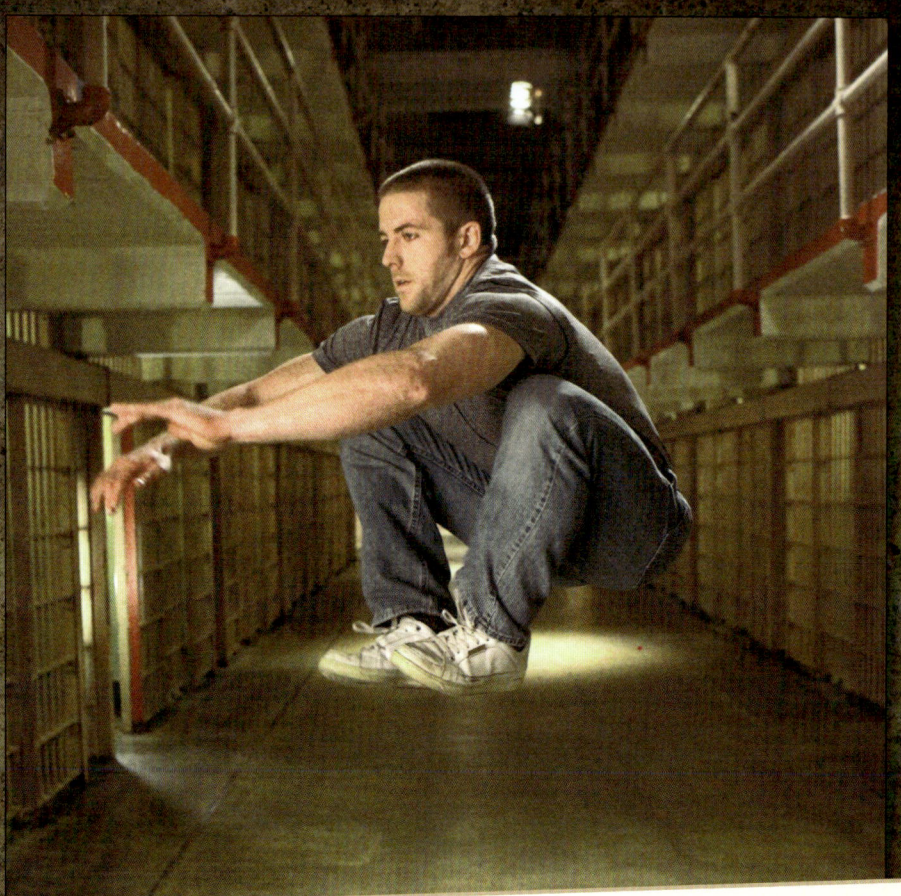

ON LEG WORK:

It's a bodybuilding myth that muscles on the opposite side of a limb always work against each other. In many cases, they work together. When you squat or run, the quadriceps and hamstrings both fire in unison to move your body through space. In medicine, this is called *Lombard's Paradox*. Forget about "isolating" your quads and hamstrings: plenty of bodyweight squats, jumps and sprints will build strong leg muscles that work in perfect harmony.

PAUL "COACH" WADE'S CONVICT CONDITIONING
Ultimate Bodyweight Training Log

DAY: _____
DATE: _____

NO.	EXERCISE	SET 1	SET 2	SET 3	SET 4	SET 5

EXTRAS:

COMMENTS:

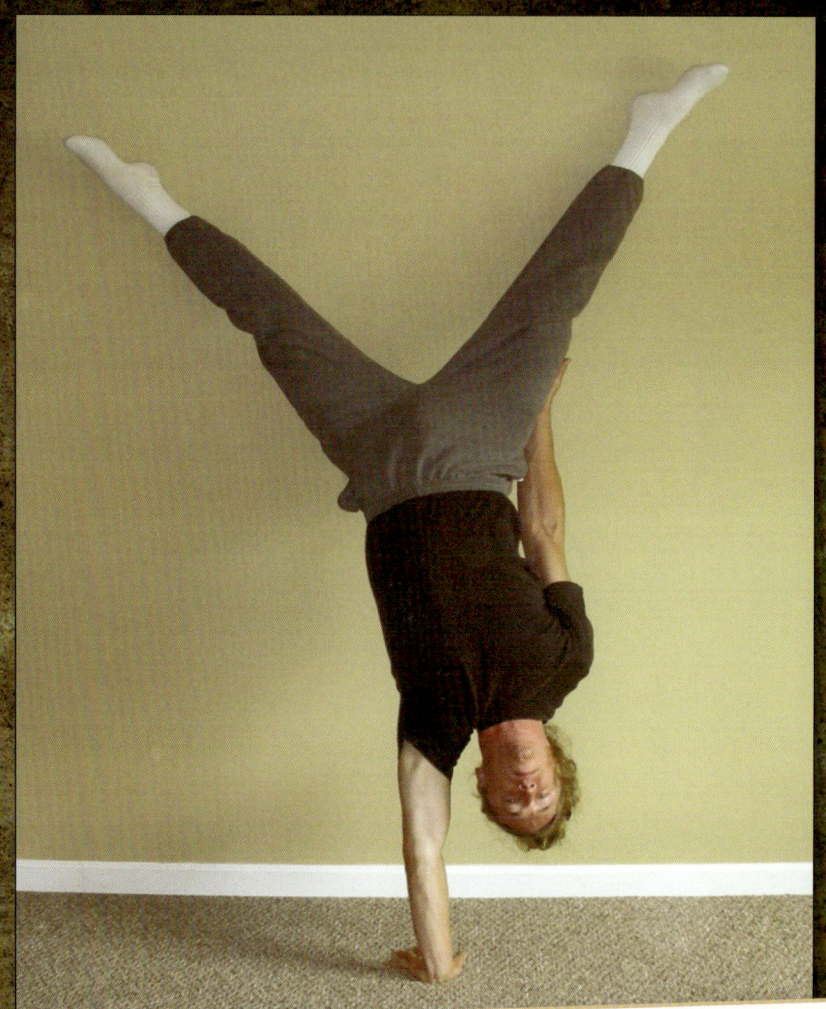

On Logan Christopher:

One of the truly great advocates of bodyweight training in the modern era is Logan Christopher. Still a young guy, Logan is known for being a strongman and hand-balancer, and has probably done more to promote handstand training than any other athlete in history. Logan can hold a perfect bridge for over ten minutes, and this ability was one of the things that made him a national calisthenics champion in 2008. Try it if you dare!

PAUL "COACH" WADE'S CONVICT CONDITIONING
Ultimate Bodyweight Training Log

DAY: _____

DATE: _____

NO.	EXERCISE	SET 1	SET 2	SET 3	SET 4	SET 5

EXTRAS:

COMMENTS:

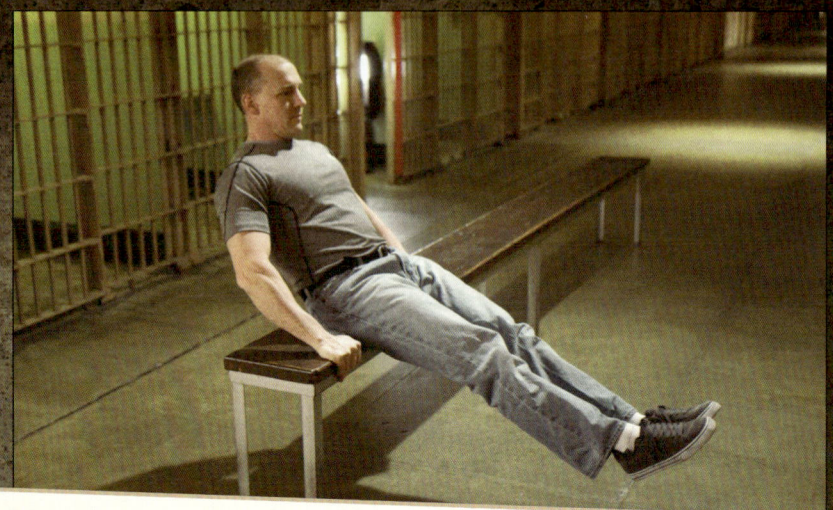

KNEE TUCKS RECORD:

One of the all-time classic midsection exercises is the simple *knee tuck*. The incredible Alicia Weber is on tape performing 401 consecutive knee tucks. What is perhaps more amazing is that this record was Weber's *seventh* record attempt of the day, and third world record performance. She had already broken the previous knee tuck and weighted knee tuck records a few hours before!

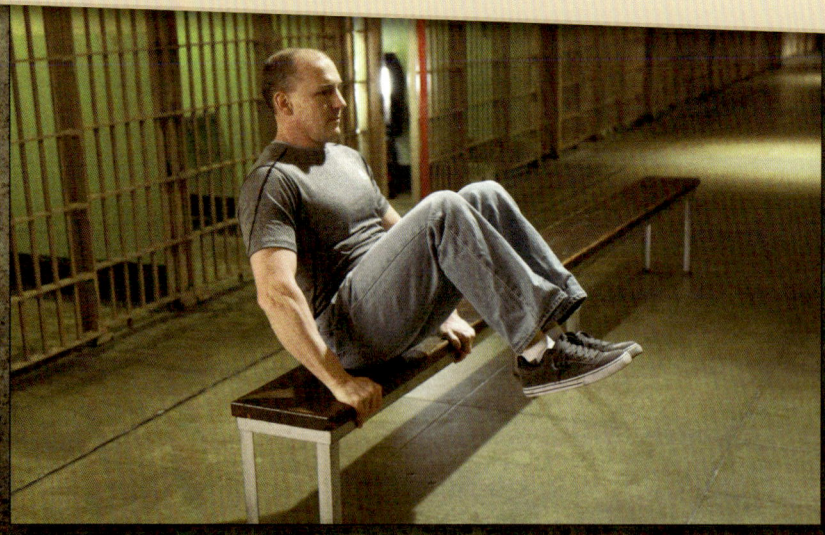

CONVICT CONDITIONING — Ultimate Bodyweight Training Log

DAY: _____

DATE: _____

NO.	EXERCISE	SET 1	SET 2	SET 3	SET 4	SET 5

EXTRAS:

COMMENTS:

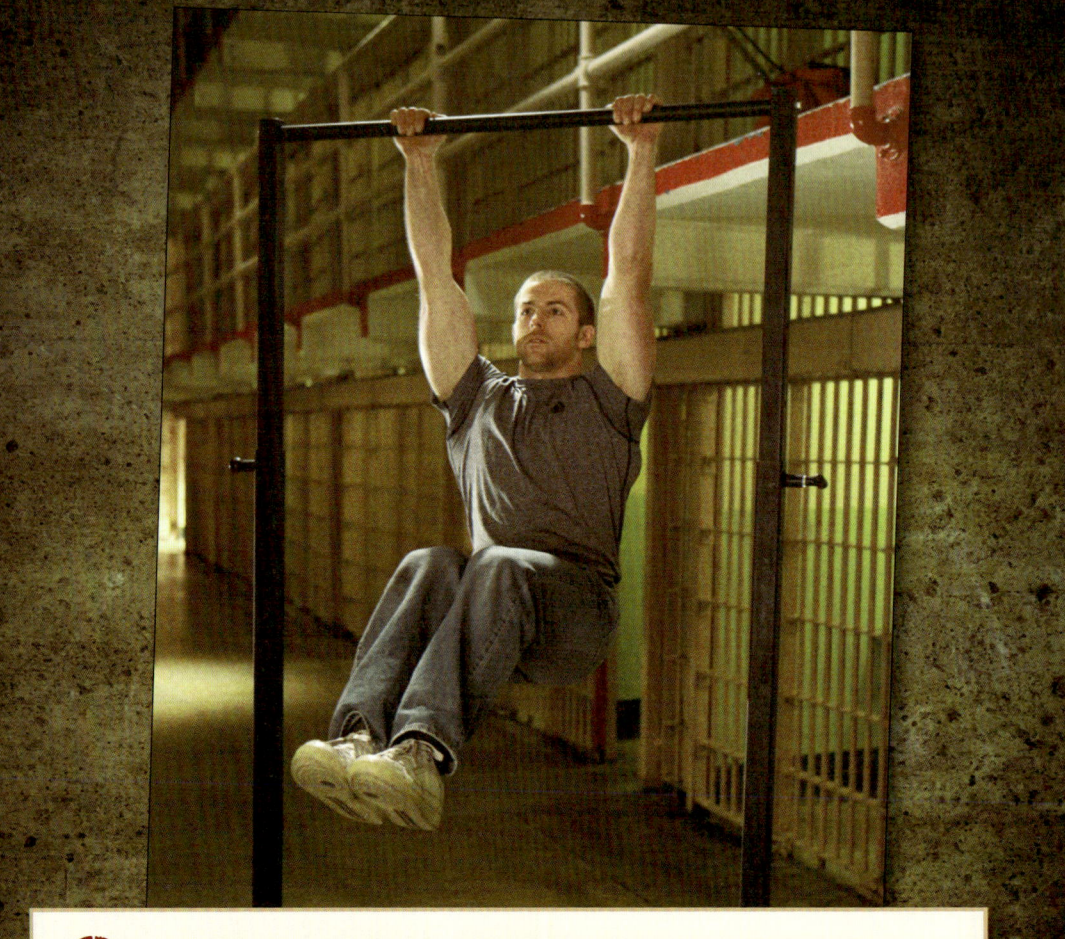

ON BRACING AND RELAXING:

Many bodyweight athletes are unsure whether they should approach their exercises braced hard, or loose and relaxed. The answer is—*it depends*. Being braced increases your strength, but too much bodily tension during a high rep set will drain your energy. If the exercise you are doing is new and difficult, and you'll be performing around six reps or less, brace yourself. If you are repping for double figures (or more) and looking to beat your PR, try not to hold any excess tension in the parts of the body that aren't moving.

PAUL "COACH" WADE'S CONVICT CONDITIONING ULTIMATE BODYWEIGHT TRAINING LOG

DAY: _____
DATE: _____

NO.	EXERCISE	SET 1	SET 2	SET 3	SET 4	SET 5

EXTRAS:

COMMENTS:

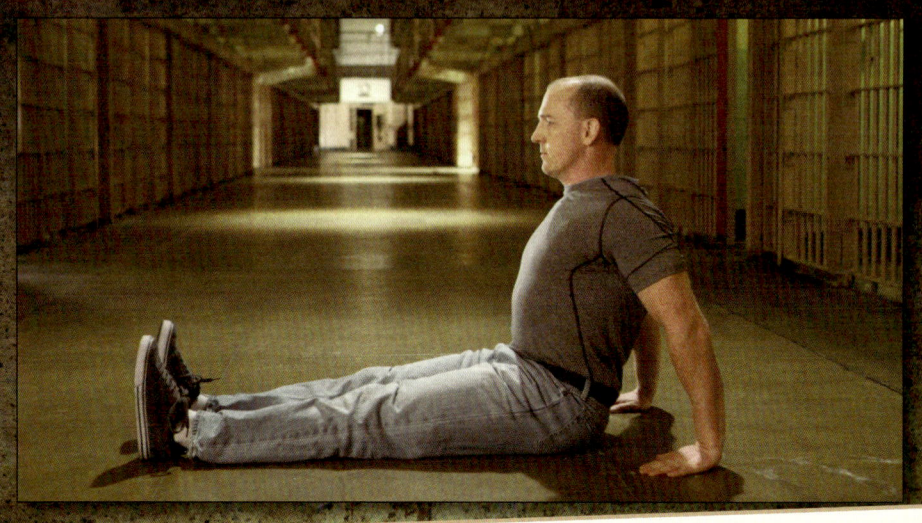

ON HAMSTRING WORK:

The best training for the back of the thighs isn't the pathetic leg curl movement—it's bridging. Bridging activates the leg biceps from both ends, the hips and knees, and brings the weight of the body into play. To set your hamstrings alight, try 4 sets of 25 strict straight bridges, followed by some explosive sprints. This workout will bulk up stubborn hamstrings in no time. Be prepared for a painful anatomy lesson the next day.

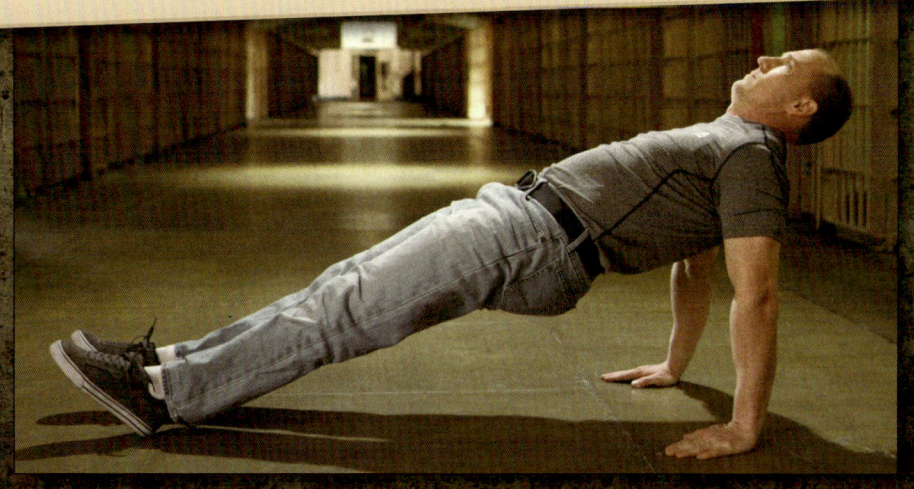

CONVICT CONDITIONING — Ultimate Bodyweight TRAINING LOG

DAY: _____

DATE: _____

NO.	EXERCISE	SET 1	SET 2	SET 3	SET 4	SET 5

EXTRAS:

COMMENTS:

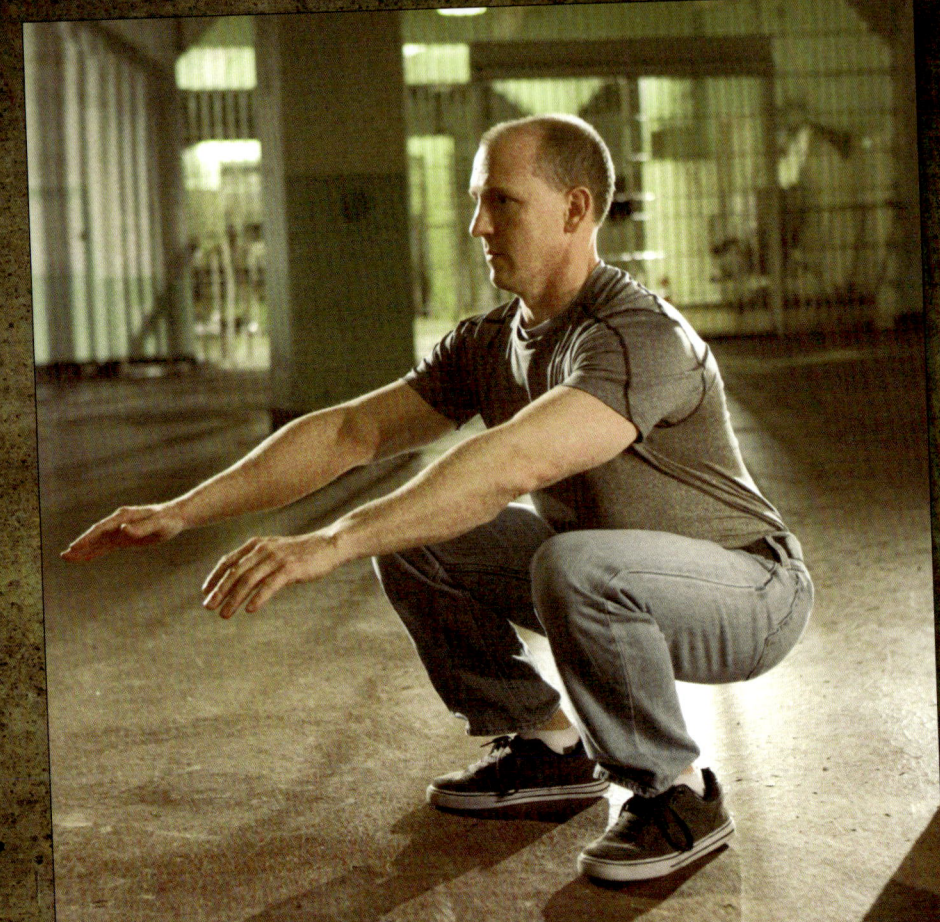

On Bodyweight Squats:

Part of the art of bodyweight squatting is about learning to lead with the *hips*, rather than the *knees*. When you squat, visualize sitting back into a chair, rather than bowing forward and bending the knees. Keeping your squats *hip-led* not only makes the exercise easier, it also takes excess pressure off the knees.

PAUL "COACH" WADE'S CONVICT CONDITIONING — Ultimate Bodyweight Training Log

DAY: _____

DATE: _____

NO.	EXERCISE	SET 1	SET 2	SET 3	SET 4	SET 5

EXTRAS:

COMMENTS:

ON LOCATION:

Convicts are often forced to limit their training to their cells or the prison yard. But bodyweight athletes beyond the bars have much more freedom. Why not train *outside* once in a while? Without the need for gym equipment, you can turn the whole world into your gym. New York City is Al Kavadlo's playground!

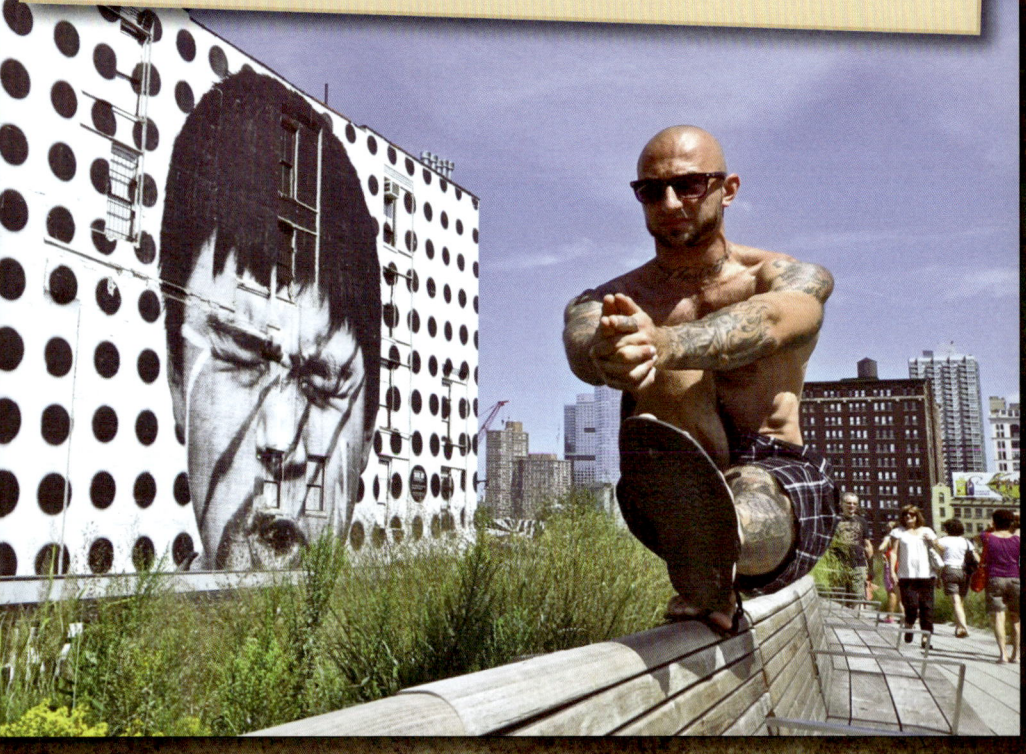

PAUL "COACH" WADE'S CONVICT CONDITIONING — ULTIMATE BODYWEIGHT TRAINING LOG

DAY: _____

DATE: _____

NO.	EXERCISE	SET 1	SET 2	SET 3	SET 4	SET 5

EXTRAS:

COMMENTS:

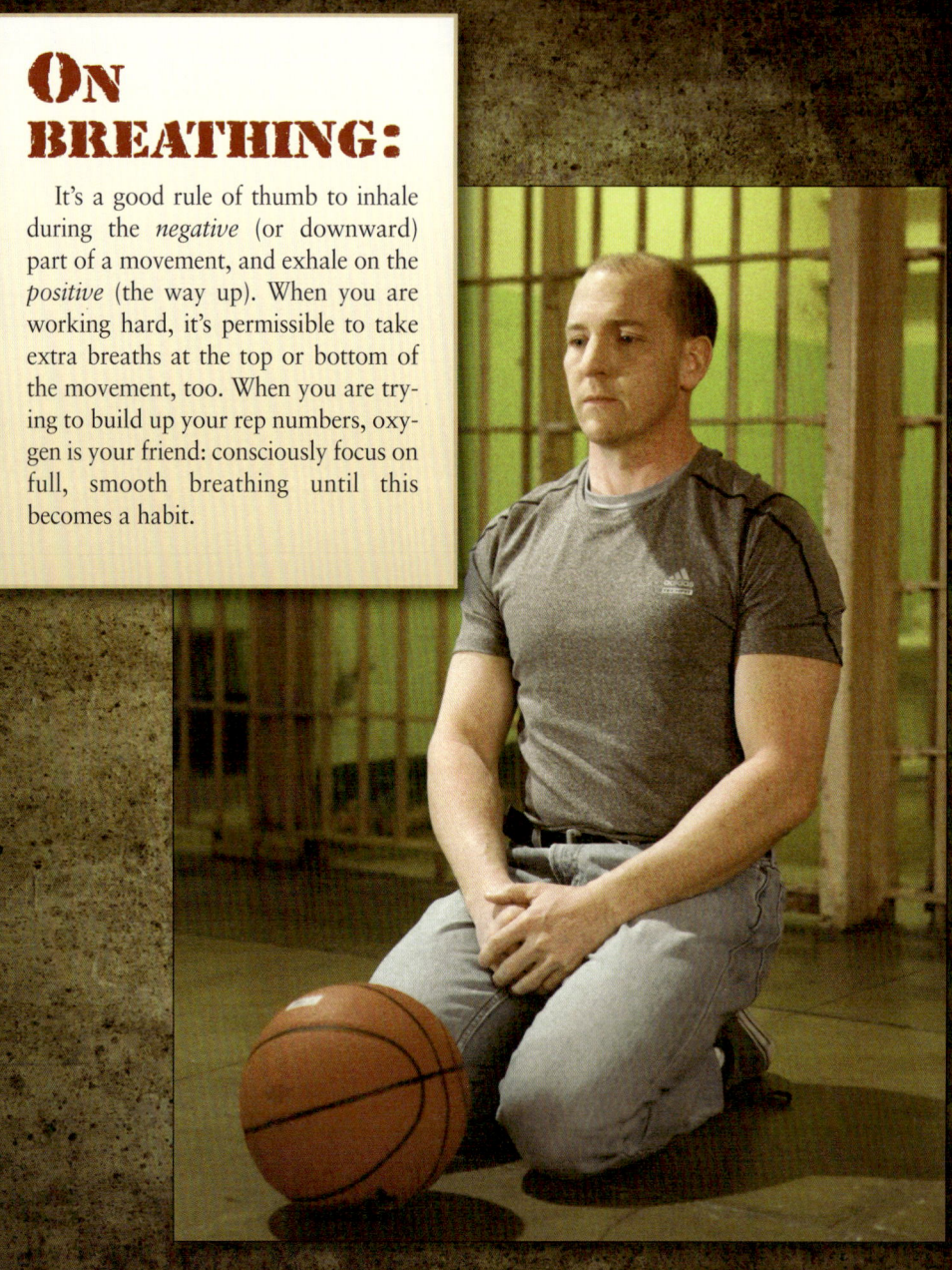

ON BREATHING:

It's a good rule of thumb to inhale during the *negative* (or downward) part of a movement, and exhale on the *positive* (the way up). When you are working hard, it's permissible to take extra breaths at the top or bottom of the movement, too. When you are trying to build up your rep numbers, oxygen is your friend: consciously focus on full, smooth breathing until this becomes a habit.

PAUL "COACH" WADE'S CONVICT CONDITIONING — Ultimate Bodyweight Training Log

DAY: _____

DATE: _____

NO.	EXERCISE	SET 1	SET 2	SET 3	SET 4	SET 5

EXTRAS:

COMMENTS:

One-arm handstand pushup record:

In 2006 the amazing Yury Tikhonovich shocked the world by performing 12 one-arm handstand pushups, from an elbow lever. This was no one-off freak feat, either; now in his 40's, Yury performs the same exhausting feat almost daily as a part of his cabaret act.

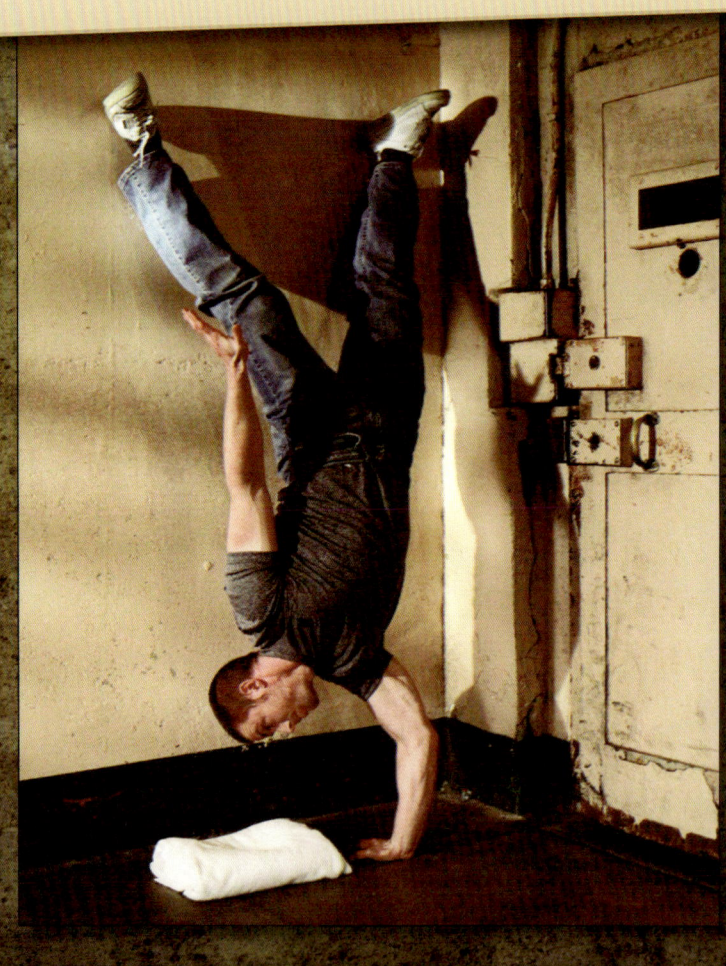

PAUL "COACH" WADE'S CONVICT CONDITIONING — Ultimate Bodyweight Training Log

71

DAY: _____

DATE: _____

NO.	EXERCISE	SET 1	SET 2	SET 3	SET 4	SET 5

EXTRAS:

COMMENTS:

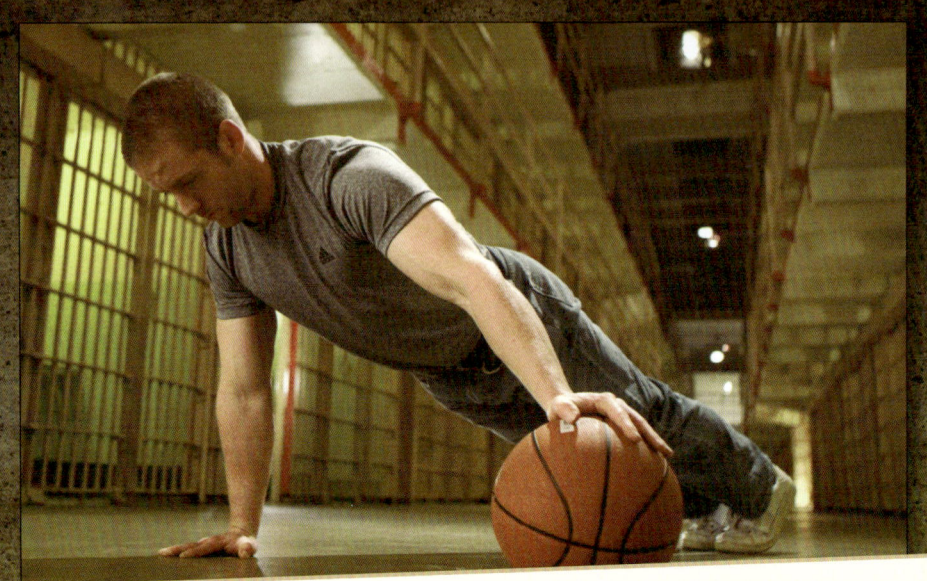

ON MOVEMENT FAMILIES:

In old school calisthenics, an exercise should never be thought of as just a single movement. Each exercise belongs to a whole "family" of movements, some of which are very easy, some of which are damn near impossible. Pushups, for example can be done at different angles, with different ranges of motion, with two-arms, one-arm or with asymmetrical arms. Every exercise in the world belongs to a similar "family hierarchy".

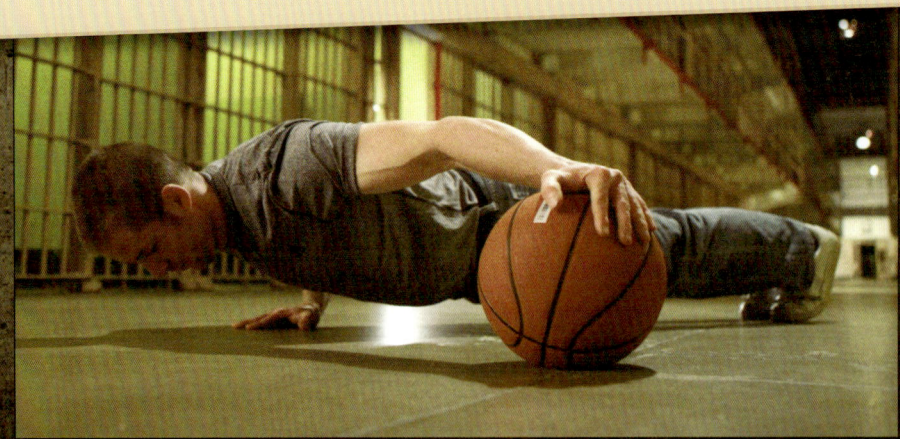

PAUL "COACH" WADE'S CONVICT CONDITIONING ULTIMATE BODYWEIGHT TRAINING LOG

DAY: _____

DATE: _____

NO.	EXERCISE	SET 1	SET 2	SET 3	SET 4	SET 5

EXTRAS:

COMMENTS:

On Abbreviated Training:

When it comes to bodyweight strength training, it's a mistake to think that more exercises will make for a better program. Pouring all your effort and focus into a handful of "big" exercises will give you better results over the long-term. Some inmates I knew spent years and years just working on pushups, pullups and one-leg squats and they gained freaky strength as a result.

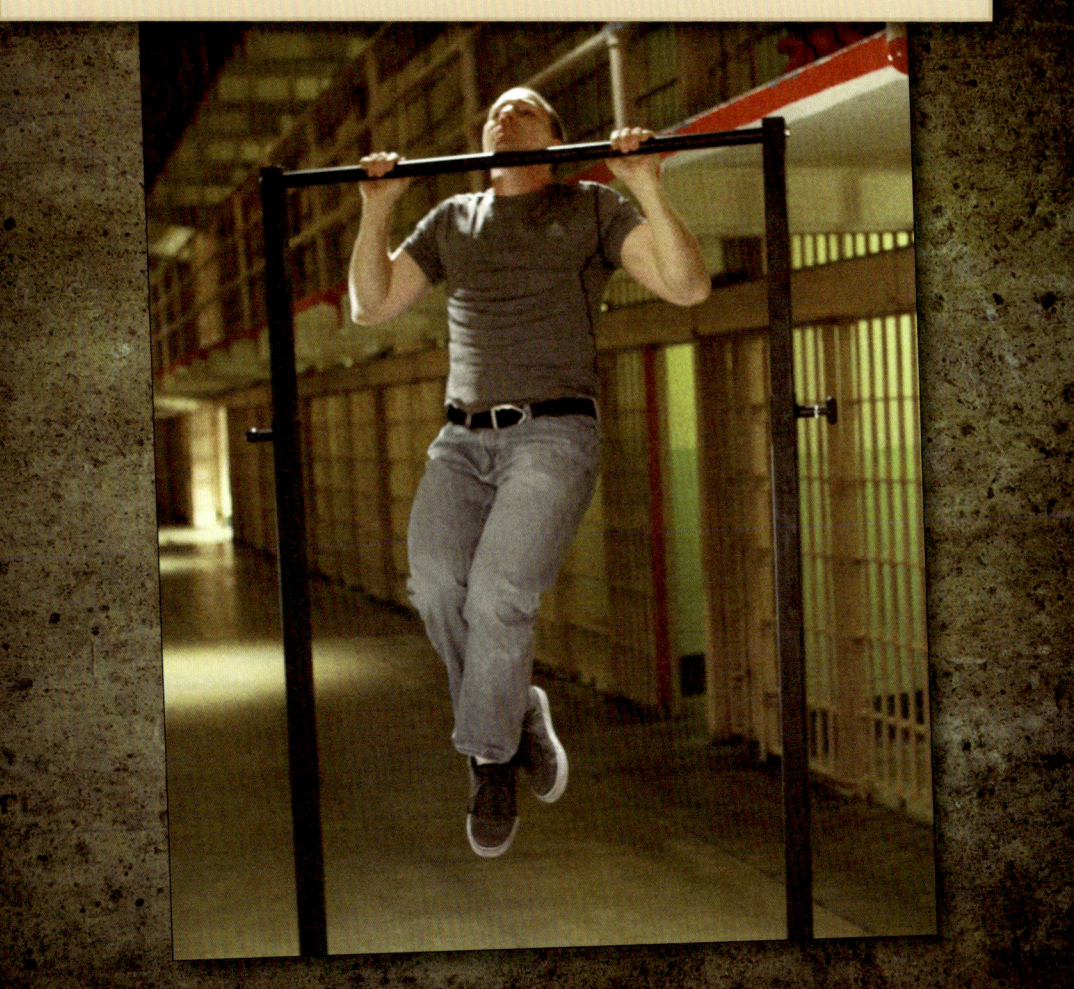

PAUL "COACH" WADE'S CONVICT CONDITIONING — ULTIMATE BODYWEIGHT TRAINING LOG

DAY: _____

DATE: _____

NO.	EXERCISE	SET 1	SET 2	SET 3	SET 4	SET 5

EXTRAS:

COMMENTS:

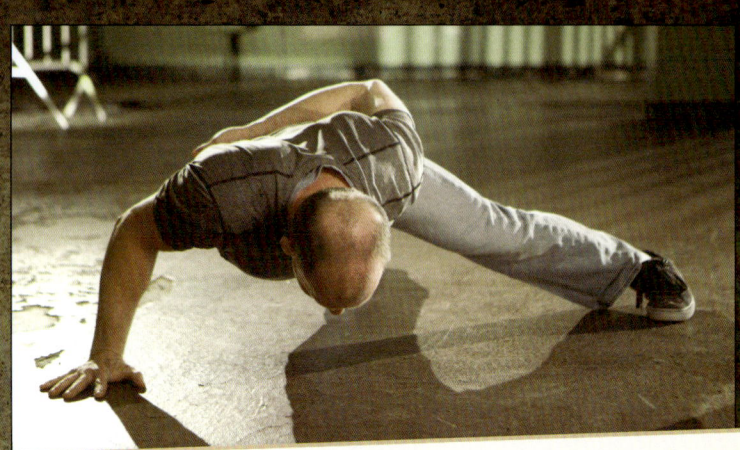

ON STABILIZATION STRENGTH:

Most gyms are full of units and machines which encourage trainees to sit or lie down while training. This is a bad trend: it eliminates the need to keep the body *stabilized*. Stabilizing yourself strengthens the network of muscles which criss-cross the trunk. To improve your stabilization strength, practice some exercises (like pushups) with just one working arm or leg, or go "gecko-style" on pushups or bridges by using one arm and the opposite leg.

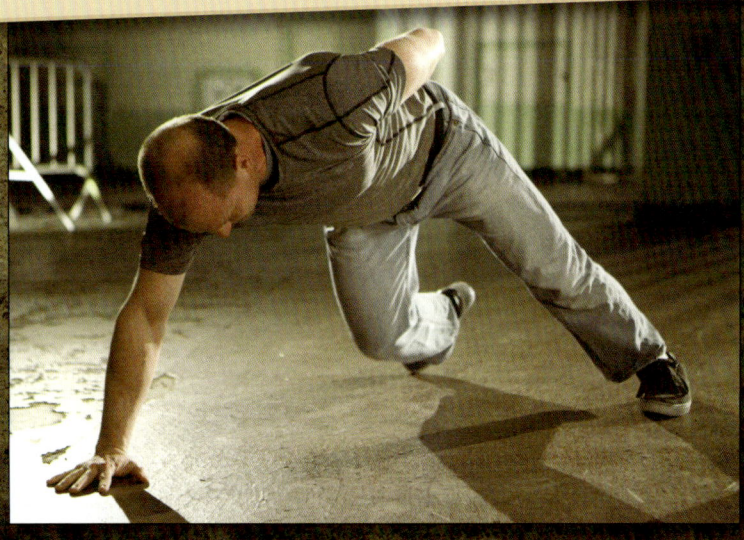

PAUL "COACH" WADE'S CONVICT CONDITIONING
ULTIMATE BODYWEIGHT TRAINING LOG

DAY: _____
DATE: _____

NO.	EXERCISE	SET 1	SET 2	SET 3	SET 4	SET 5

EXTRAS:

COMMENTS:

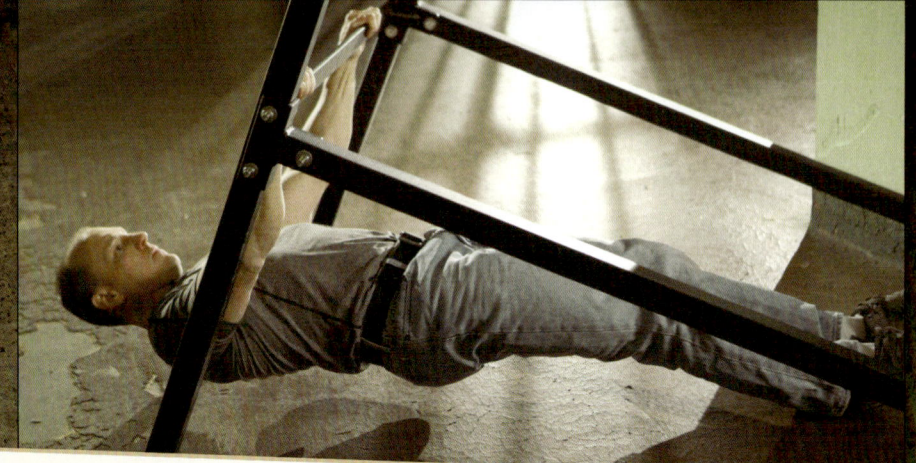

WEBER'S PULLUP EXCELLENCE:

Guys who bitch and moan when I tell them to build up their reps on the horizontal pull should maybe take a lesson from the ladies. In 2011 American girl Alicia Weber officially performed 75 pullups in three minutes (while you were still working out where the pullup bar was). In case you think a mere three minutes burnt her out, she also managed 432 pullups in just half an hour.

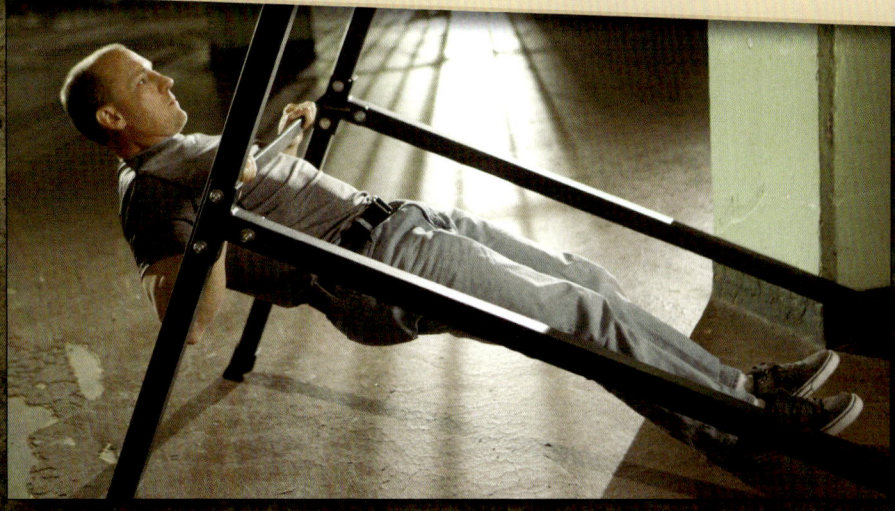

CONVICT CONDITIONING — Ultimate Bodyweight TRAINING LOG

DAY: _____
DATE: _____

NO.	EXERCISE	SET 1	SET 2	SET 3	SET 4	SET 5

EXTRAS:

COMMENTS:

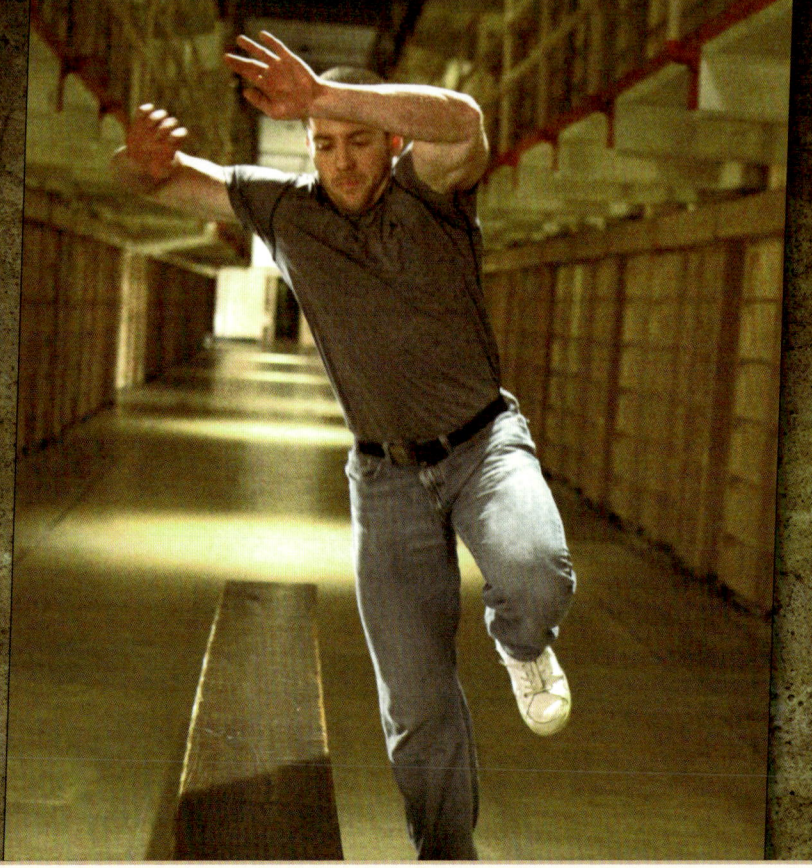

ON SURVIVAL ATHLETICS:

Prisoners don't think in terms of "cardio" when they do higher rep workouts. Instead, they think in terms of *survival athletics*. Ditch the stationary bike or rowing machine, and pick functional bodyweight movements when you want to sweat. Use your body to get down and get up again in different ways, always moving as fast as you can. Try mixing up a ten minute circuit of burpees, speed get-ups lying on your front or back, kip-ups, ducks and jumps.

PAUL "COACH" WADE'S CONVICT CONDITIONING — Ultimate Bodyweight Training Log

81

DAY: _____

DATE: _____

NO.	EXERCISE	SET 1	SET 2	SET 3	SET 4	SET 5

EXTRAS:

COMMENTS:

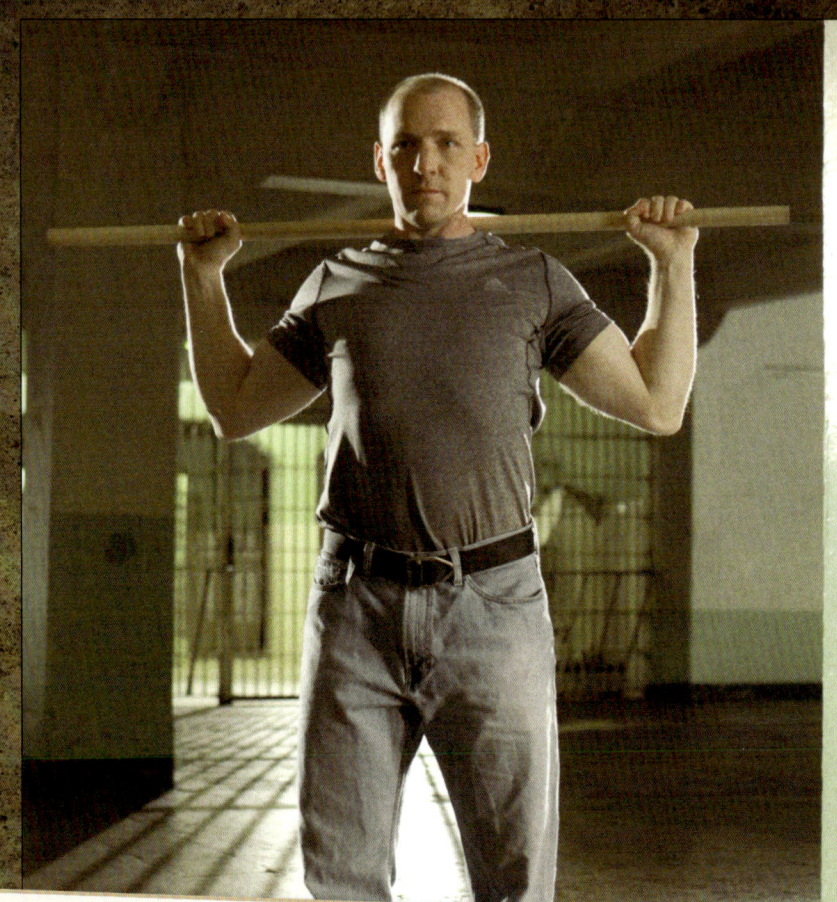

On Warming up:

Warming up is a crucial part of training, but many athletes are taught to overdo it. If your warm ups are detrimentally affecting your performance on your "work" sets, then you are doing too much. For most men and women, a light warm up of joint circling followed by two or three easier variations of the exercise you are planning on working with is enough. Only add more than this if you really need to: maybe if you are cold, carrying an injury, etc.

PAUL "COACH" WADE'S CONVICT CONDITIONING ULTIMATE BODYWEIGHT TRAINING LOG

83

DAY: _____

DATE: _____

NO.	EXERCISE	SET 1	SET 2	SET 3	SET 4	SET 5

EXTRAS:

COMMENTS:

MORE ON LEG TRAINING:

Heavy barbell squats and leg presses cause stiffness over time. Once you can perform a full one-leg squat, don't get stuck in a rut of adding more and more weight. Now is the time to explore more *useful* lower body qualities: speed, balance, power, endurance, and agility. What's the point of a huge squat if you get out of breath climbing stairs? Run hills, jump and leap, sprint, kick the heavy bag!

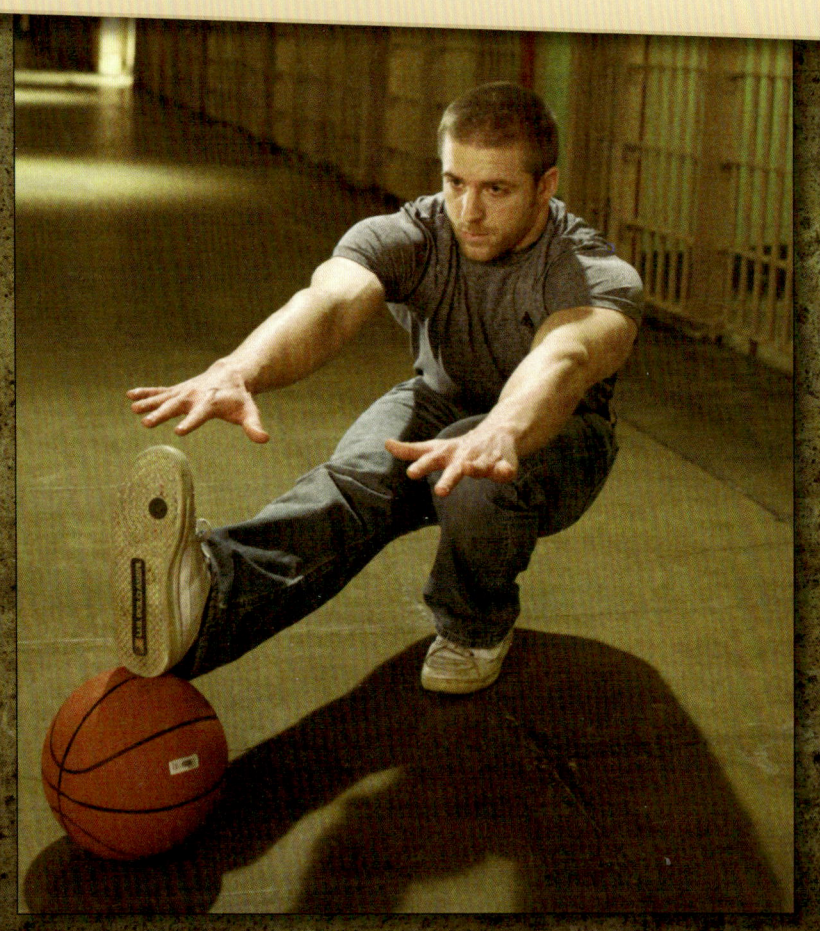

PAUL "COACH" WADE'S CONVICT CONDITIONING — ULTIMATE BODYWEIGHT TRAINING LOG

DAY: _____
DATE: _____

NO.	EXERCISE	SET 1	SET 2	SET 3	SET 4	SET 5

EXTRAS:

COMMENTS:

On Bodyweight Hypers:

A lot of athletes who want to give their lower backs some load-free therapy or conditioning head over to the hyperextension unit in the gym. But prisoners have long understood that you can perform reverse hypers without any equipment at all. Get into a solid headstand and, keeping the legs together and extended, smoothly lower your feet towards the floor, then lift back up. Bodyweight hypers performed for high repetitions have a powerful rejuvenating and healing effect on battered lower backs.

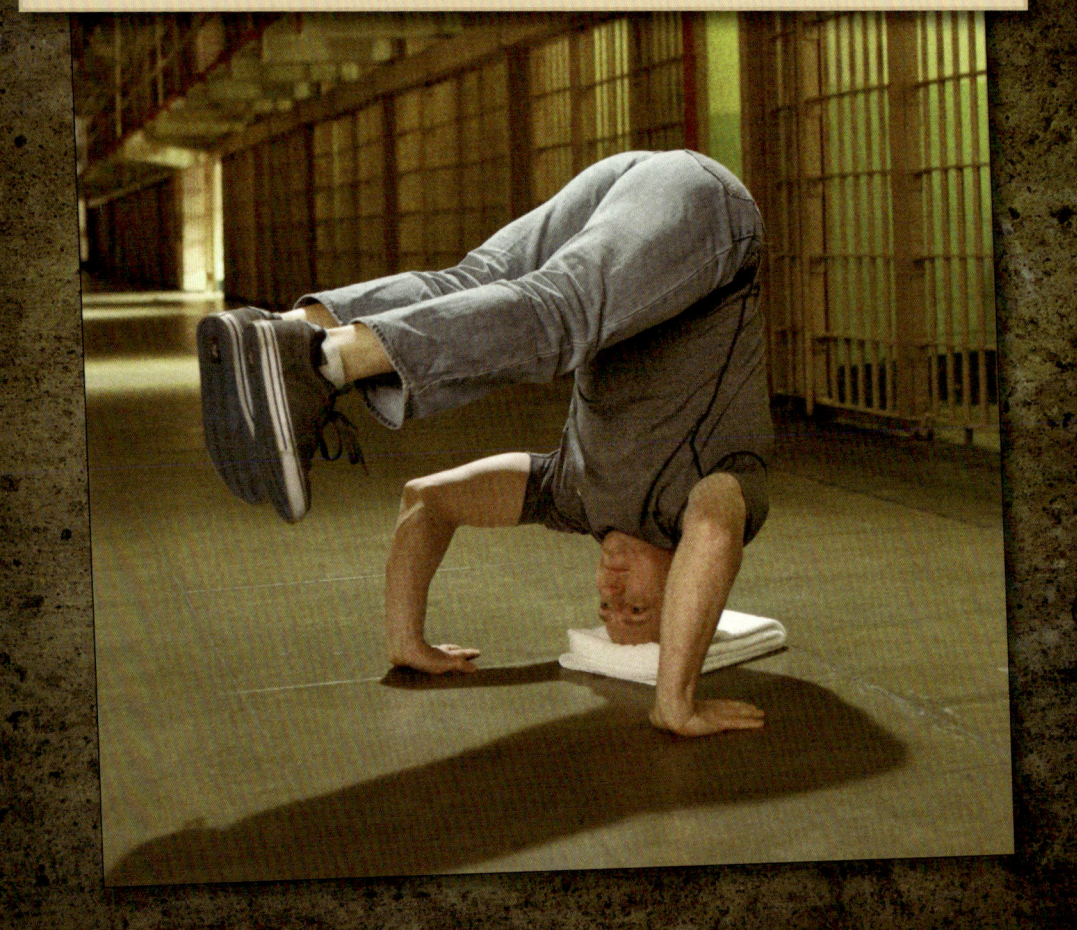

PAUL "COACH" WADE'S CONVICT CONDITIONING

ULTIMATE BODYWEIGHT TRAINING LOG

DAY: _____
DATE: _____

NO.	EXERCISE	SET 1	SET 2	SET 3	SET 4	SET 5

EXTRAS:

COMMENTS:

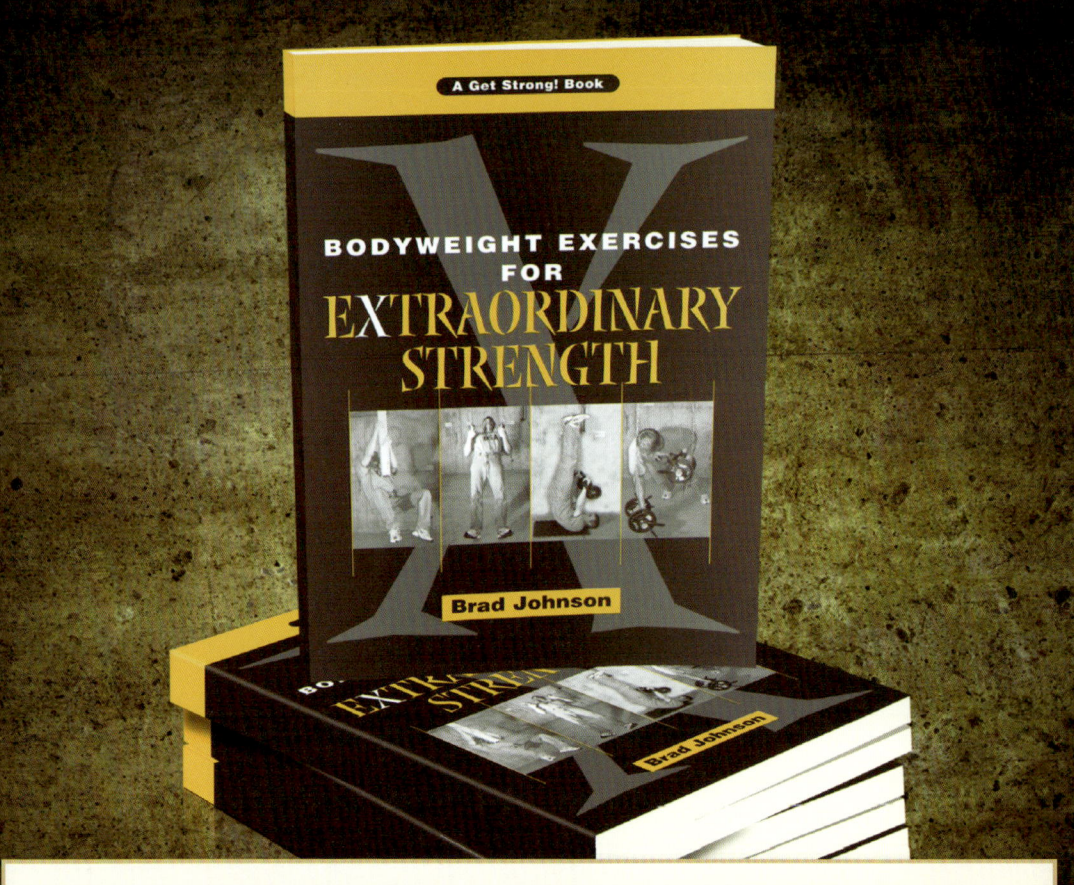

Great Bodyweight Strength Books # 3:
Bodyweight Exercises for Extraordinary Strength—Brad Johnson

Question: Why did IronMind, a world famous *equipment* manufacturer, publish a book about bodyweight training? *Answer:* Because it is possibly the best book on *real strength* ever written. When I read Brad's book, it immediately struck a nerve; Brad's approach is remarkably similar to that of my mentor, Joe Hartigen. Had he lived to read it, this would have been Joe's favorite training manual. I have told Brad that without his book, *Convict Conditioning* would never have been written.

PAUL "COACH" WADE'S CONVICT CONDITIONING
Ultimate Bodyweight Training Log

DAY: _____

DATE: _____

NO.	EXERCISE	SET 1	SET 2	SET 3	SET 4	SET 5

EXTRAS:

COMMENTS:

ON COOL DOWNS:

The idea of needing a "cool down" is a myth which originated with Victorian physical culturalists. Scientists now know that that the body doesn't really *need* a cool down: like a lion in the hunt, an athlete can go from 100% exertion to sudden inactivity with no ill effects. If you want to cool down for psychological reasons, you can do it, but there's no physical necessity. After a tough workout, I like to regain equilibrium by performing deep breathing exercises.

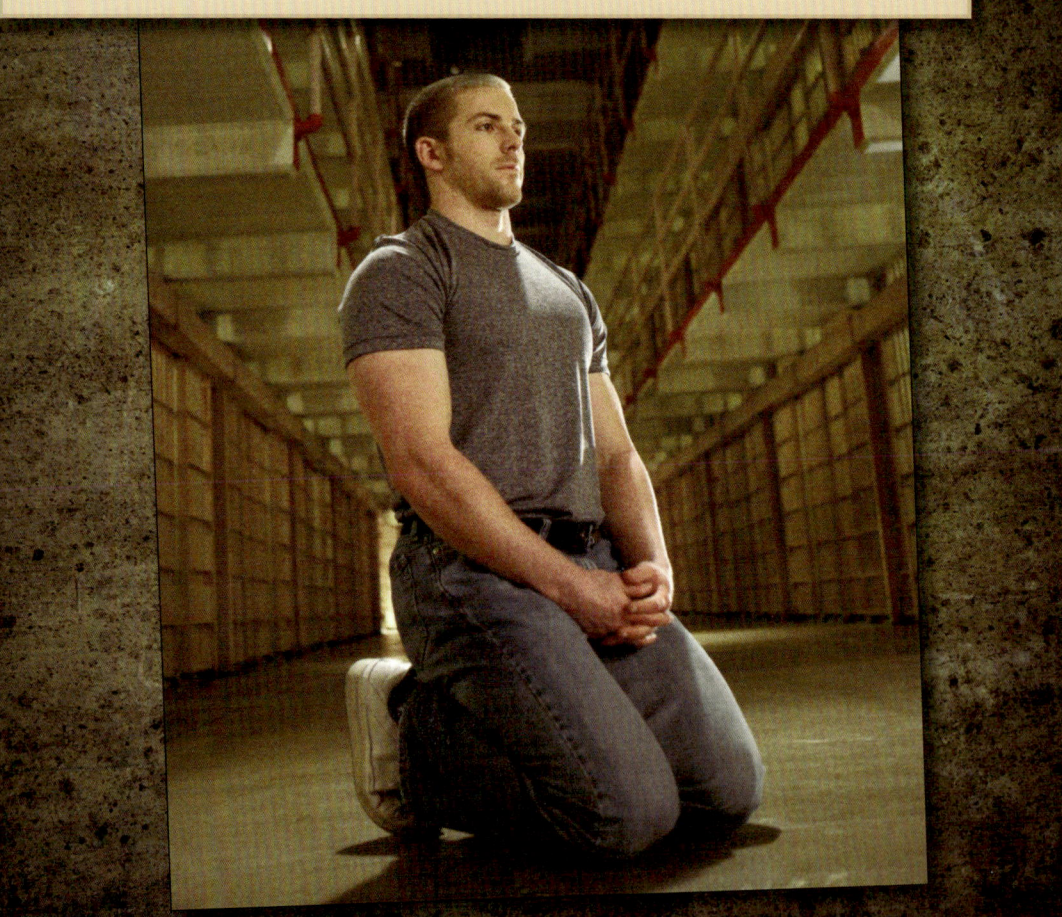

PAUL "COACH" WADE'S CONVICT CONDITIONING — Ultimate Bodyweight Training Log

DAY: _____

DATE: _____

NO.	EXERCISE	SET 1	SET 2	SET 3	SET 4	SET 5

EXTRAS:

COMMENTS:

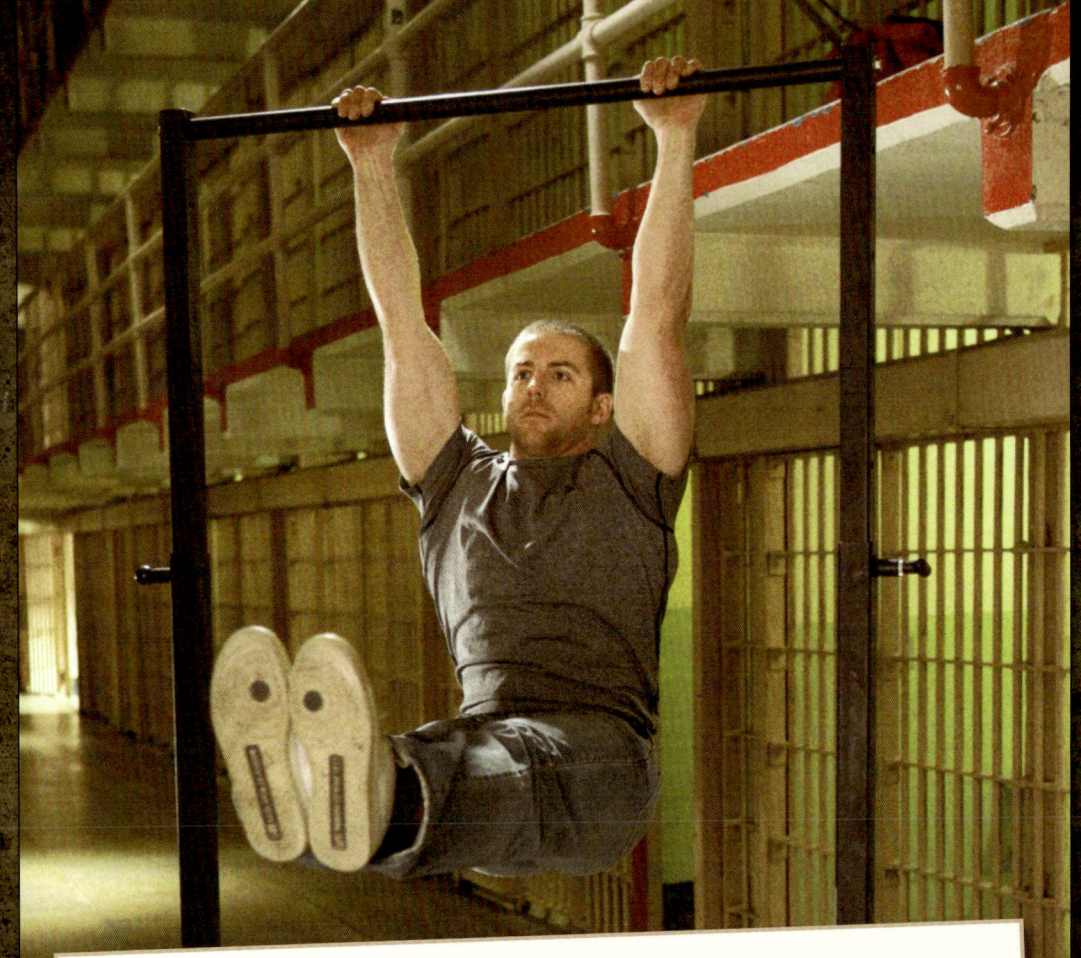

ON MIDSECTION SPECIALIZATION:

If an athlete works hard on the big exercises, the entire body gets worked as a unit, and there will be no real need for the midsection specialization workouts so loved by the fitness magazines. If you really are a midsection freak, you can get a perfect midsection workout by combining *hanging leg raises*, *bridges*, *human flags* and *spinal twists*. Those four families, worked progressively, are all any athlete would ever need for a superhuman gut and waist.

Paul "Coach" Wade's CONVICT CONDITIONING Ultimate Bodyweight TRAINING LOG

DAY: _____

DATE: _____

NO.	EXERCISE	SET 1	SET 2	SET 3	SET 4	SET 5

EXTRAS:

COMMENTS:

ON POST-WORKOUT NUTRITION:

I'm not a big believer in the need for post-workout nutrition: in fact I think most of it is a myth made up by the supplement companies. Remember, you begin to absorb and utilize the nutrients of a food not when you eat or drink it, but only *after digestion*. Most of the athletes glugging down post-workout shakes don't need those shakes because they are *still digesting* the meals they ate before their workout. Red meat can take up to *three days* to digest!

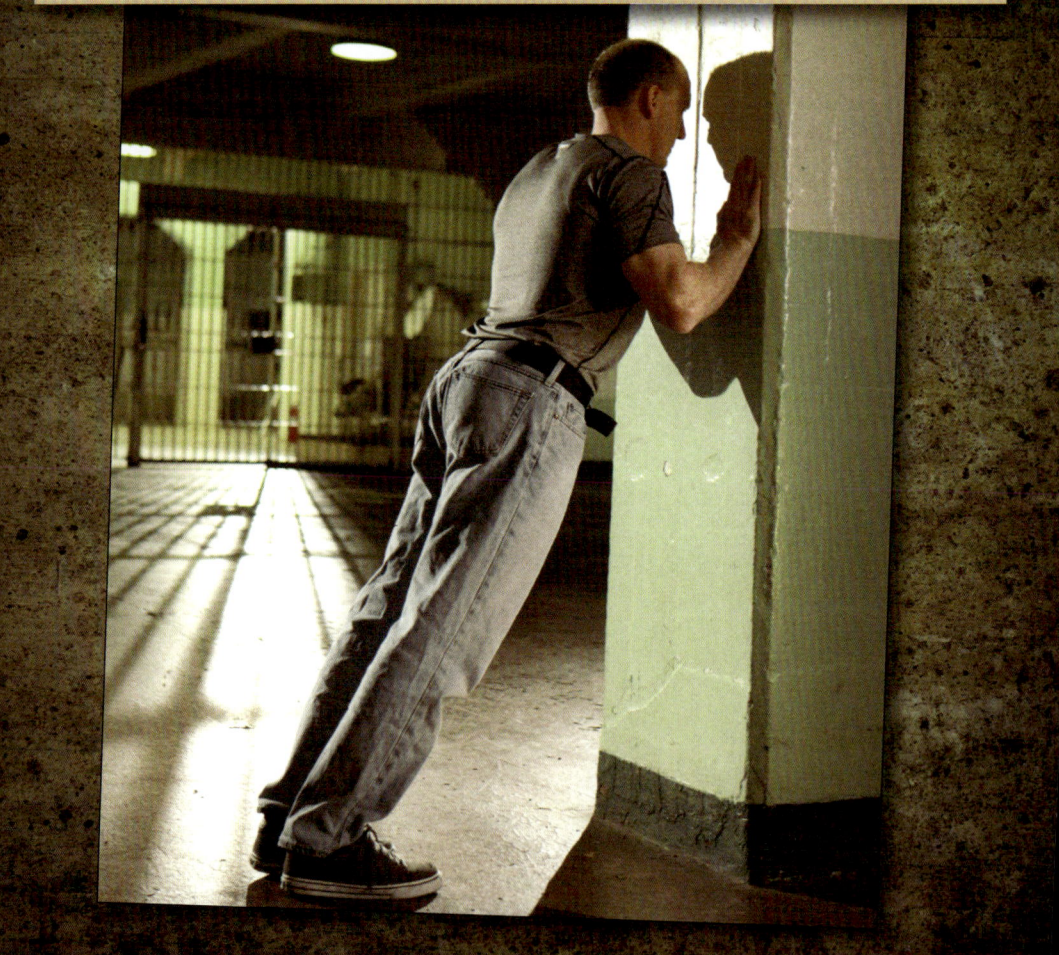

PAUL "COACH" WADE'S CONVICT CONDITIONING — Ultimate Bodyweight Training Log

DAY: _____

DATE: _____

NO.	EXERCISE	SET 1	SET 2	SET 3	SET 4	SET 5

EXTRAS:

COMMENTS:

ON SETS:

When I was a new fish, I was guilty of pumping out many dozens of daily sets in my quest for fresh strength and muscle. As I got older and wiser, I found that I progressed just as fast when I used no more than two hard sets per exercise. My muscles were fresher, I had more motivation, and I recovered quicker, too. If you want stamina you need to hit lots and lots of sets, but for power and mass more effort over fewer sets is king. Certainly anything over five sets is a waste.

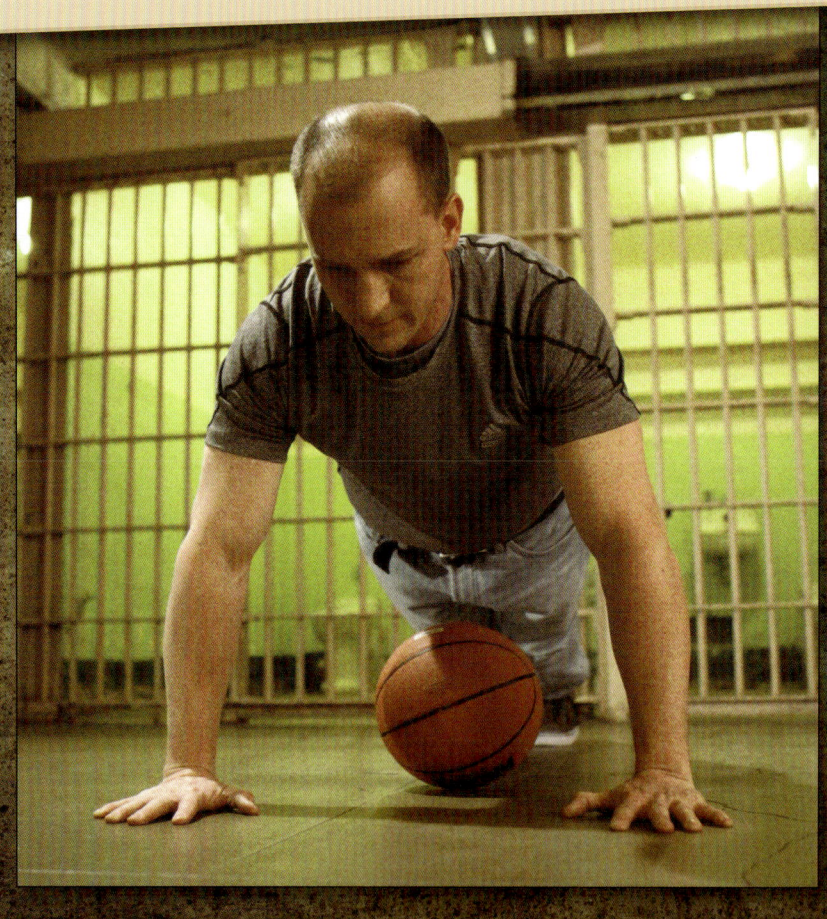

PAUL "COACH" WADE'S CONVICT CONDITIONING — Ultimate Bodyweight Training Log

DAY: _____

DATE: _____

NO.	EXERCISE	SET 1	SET 2	SET 3	SET 4	SET 5

EXTRAS:

COMMENTS:

ON KNEE SQUATS:

Knee squats are an excellent transitional exercise that can help you build the strength to dominate one-leg squats. Bend one leg so that the knee points to the floor, and lower yourself until your kneecap gently kisses the ground. Press up smoothly and without momentum. Al Kavadlo calls this exercise "shrimp squats"; Pavel Tsatsouline calls them "airborne lunges".

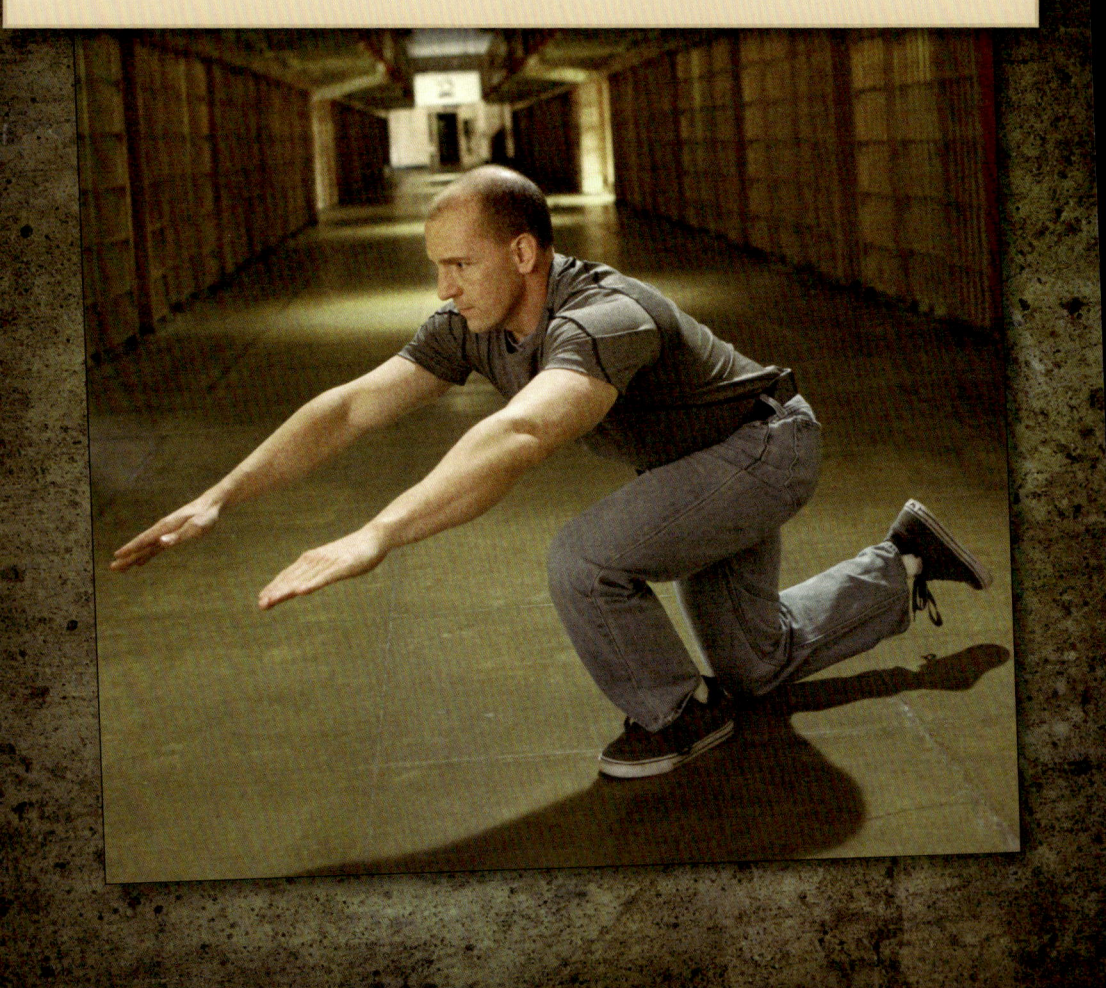

CONVICT CONDITIONING — Ultimate Bodyweight Training Log

DAY: _____

DATE: _____

NO.	EXERCISE	SET 1	SET 2	SET 3	SET 4	SET 5

EXTRAS:

COMMENTS:

ON TWISTING:

Athletes are used to *pushing* and *pulling*, but how many of them seriously *twist* as part of their workouts? Spinal twists release the shoulders, strengthen the rotator cuffs, cure back pain and tone the entire midsection. They even aid digestion. If you ain't doing them…why not?

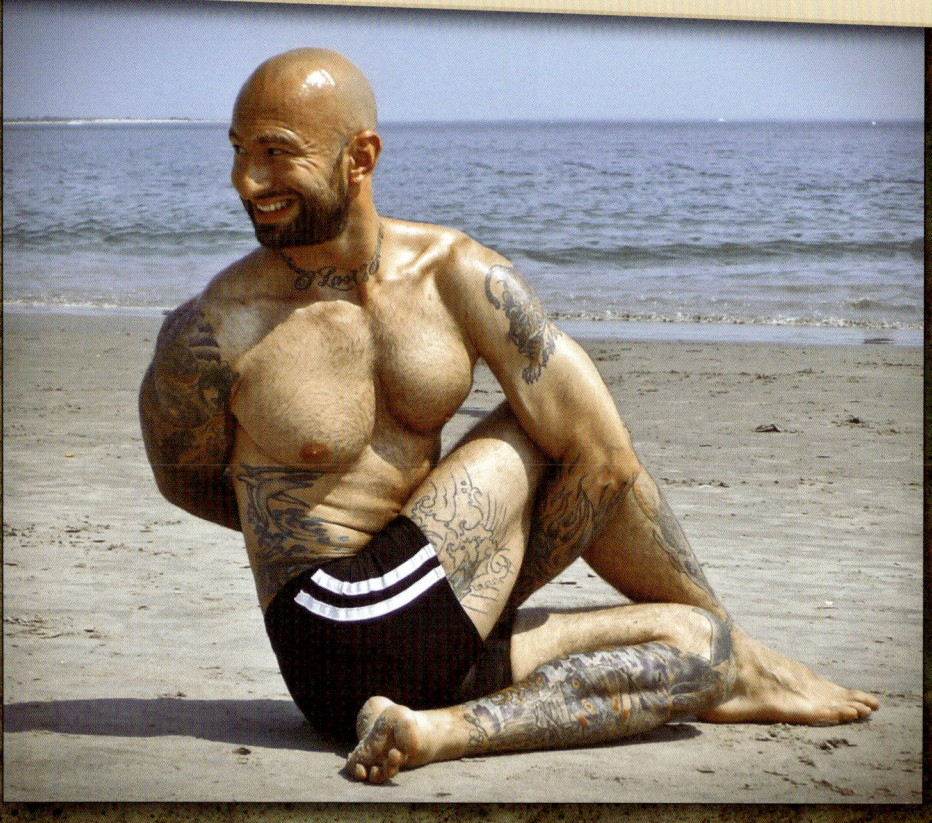

PAUL "COACH" WADE'S CONVICT CONDITIONING ULTIMATE BODYWEIGHT TRAINING LOG

101

DAY:_____

DATE:_____

NO.	EXERCISE	SET 1	SET 2	SET 3	SET 4	SET 5

EXTRAS:

COMMENTS:

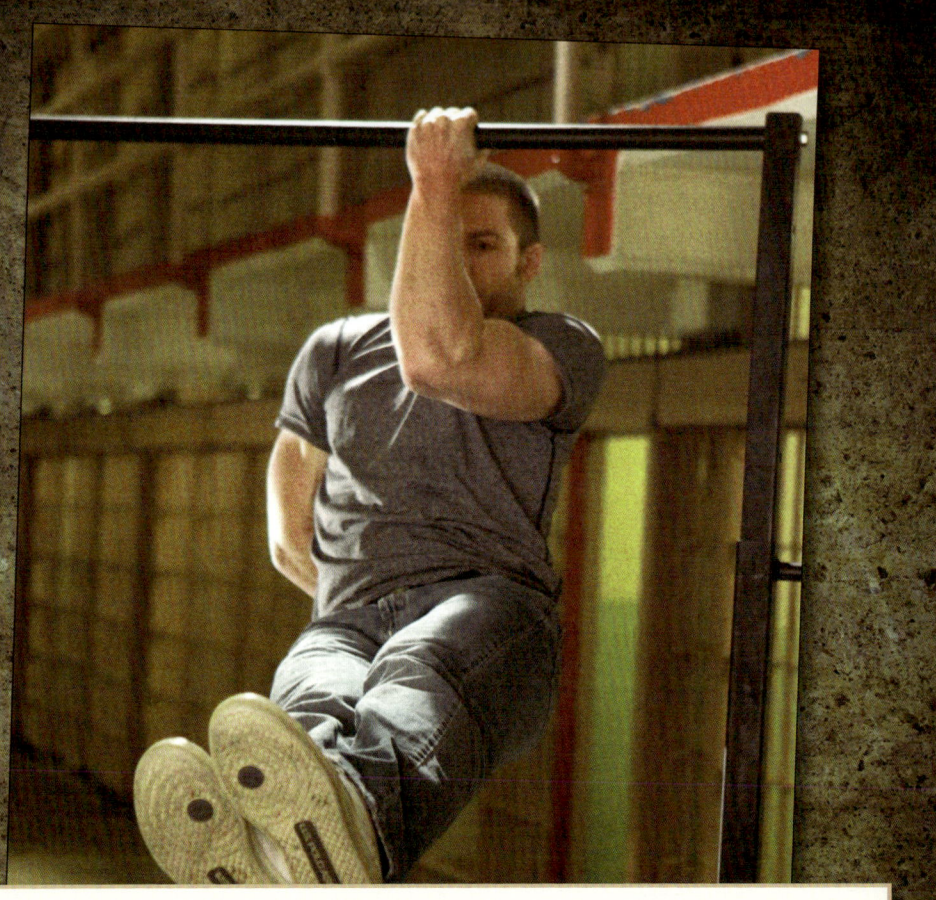

On old school calisthenics:

A lot of people ask me to define "old school calisthenics". Old school calisthenics is an *approach*: not a "system", or a "workout". The approach is simple. Pick a bodyweight exercise, and learn to do it well. As you gain ability, add reps over time. Once you hit a target number of reps, find a way to make the exercise harder. Repeat that process until you can bend steel bars.

CONVICT CONDITIONING ULTIMATE BODYWEIGHT TRAINING LOG

DAY: _____

DATE: _____

NO.	EXERCISE	SET 1	SET 2	SET 3	SET 4	SET 5

EXTRAS:

COMMENTS:

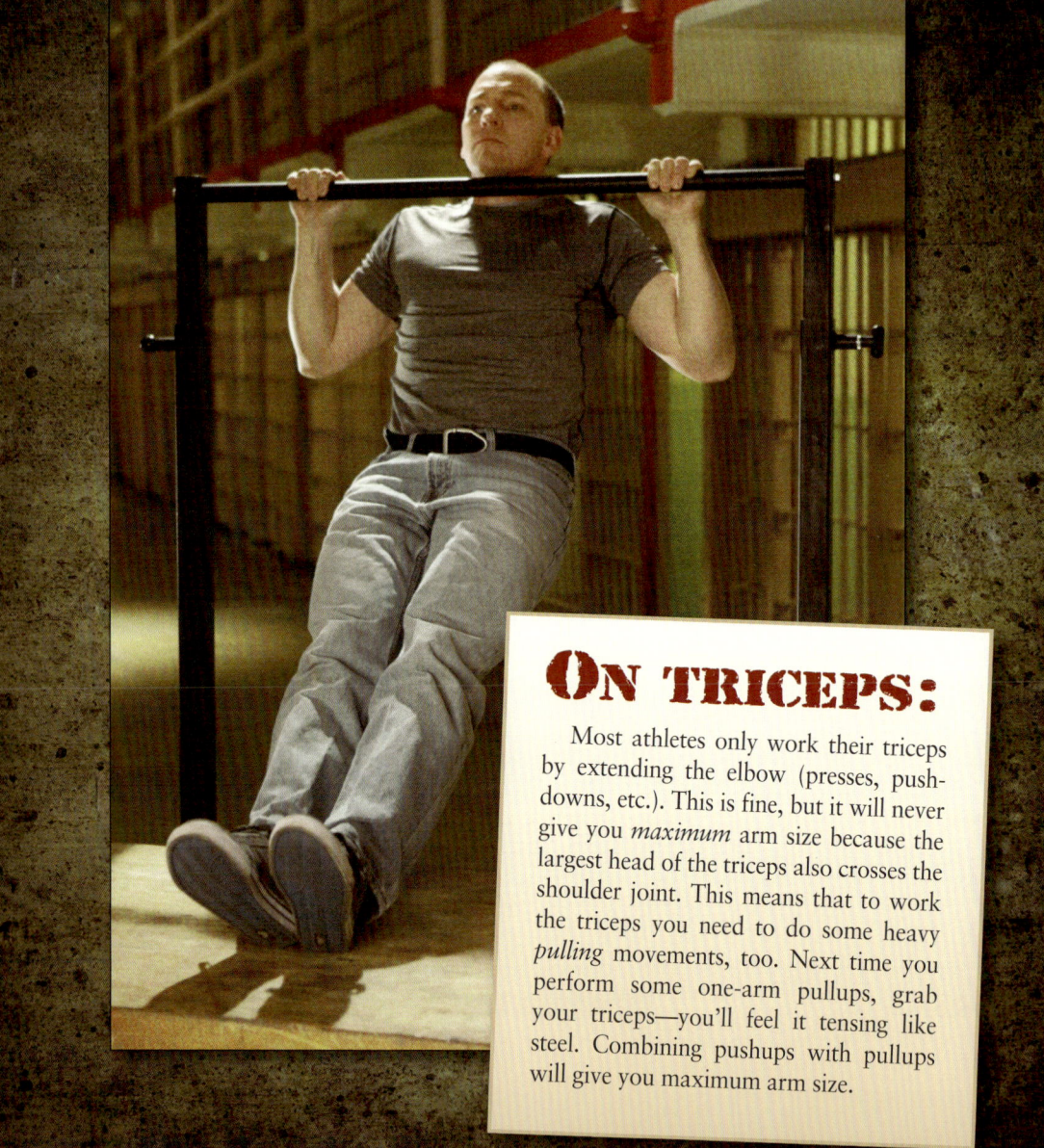

ON TRICEPS:

Most athletes only work their triceps by extending the elbow (presses, pushdowns, etc.). This is fine, but it will never give you *maximum* arm size because the largest head of the triceps also crosses the shoulder joint. This means that to work the triceps you need to do some heavy *pulling* movements, too. Next time you perform some one-arm pullups, grab your triceps—you'll feel it tensing like steel. Combining pushups with pullups will give you maximum arm size.

CONVICT CONDITIONING
PAUL "COACH" WADE'S ULTIMATE BODYWEIGHT TRAINING LOG

DAY: _____

DATE: _____

NO.	EXERCISE	SET 1	SET 2	SET 3	SET 4	SET 5

EXTRAS:

COMMENTS:

On Inverse Training:

Even if you never plan to do a single handstand pushup, every athlete should get *inverse*—upside-down—at least once a week. Being wrongside-up for a while tones the circulatory system, refreshes the organs, improves balance and sends new blood to the brain and cervical spine. Very few methods of training have so many benefits. Train right, and inverse work is also very safe. If handstands are out, try headstands or hanging inverted on the pullup bar.

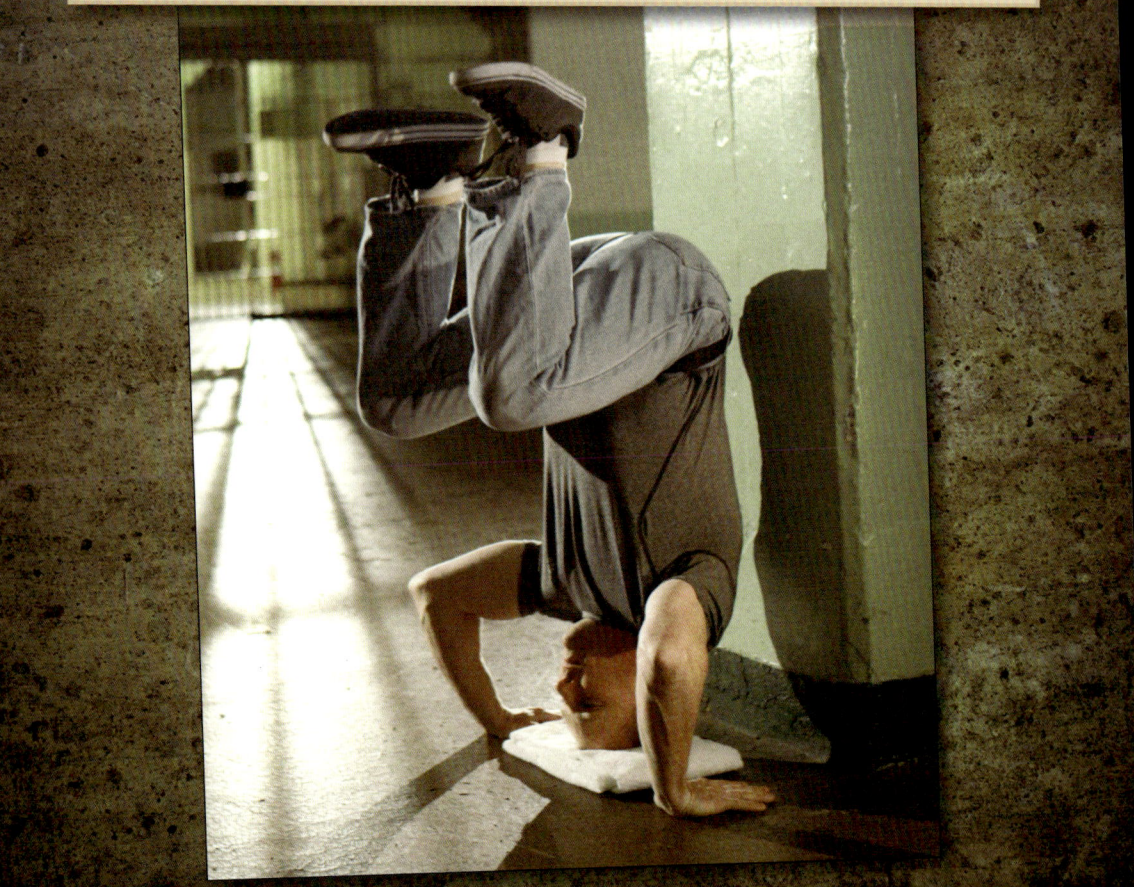

CONVICT CONDITIONING ULTIMATE BODYWEIGHT TRAINING LOG

DAY: _____
DATE: _____

NO.	EXERCISE	SET 1	SET 2	SET 3	SET 4	SET 5

EXTRAS:

COMMENTS:

On Banking Strength:

Banking strength is like banking money. Killing yourself to massively improve strength *every* workout is like trying to stick your whole paycheck into your savings every month—very soon you'll have to quit due to lack of daily funds! It's much better to cautiously add a *little* money to your savings, consistently; after a while you'll have a lot of cash saved, with very little stress. Likewise, build strength slowly and moderately workout by workout, without beating yourself up: before long, you'll have massive reserves of power.

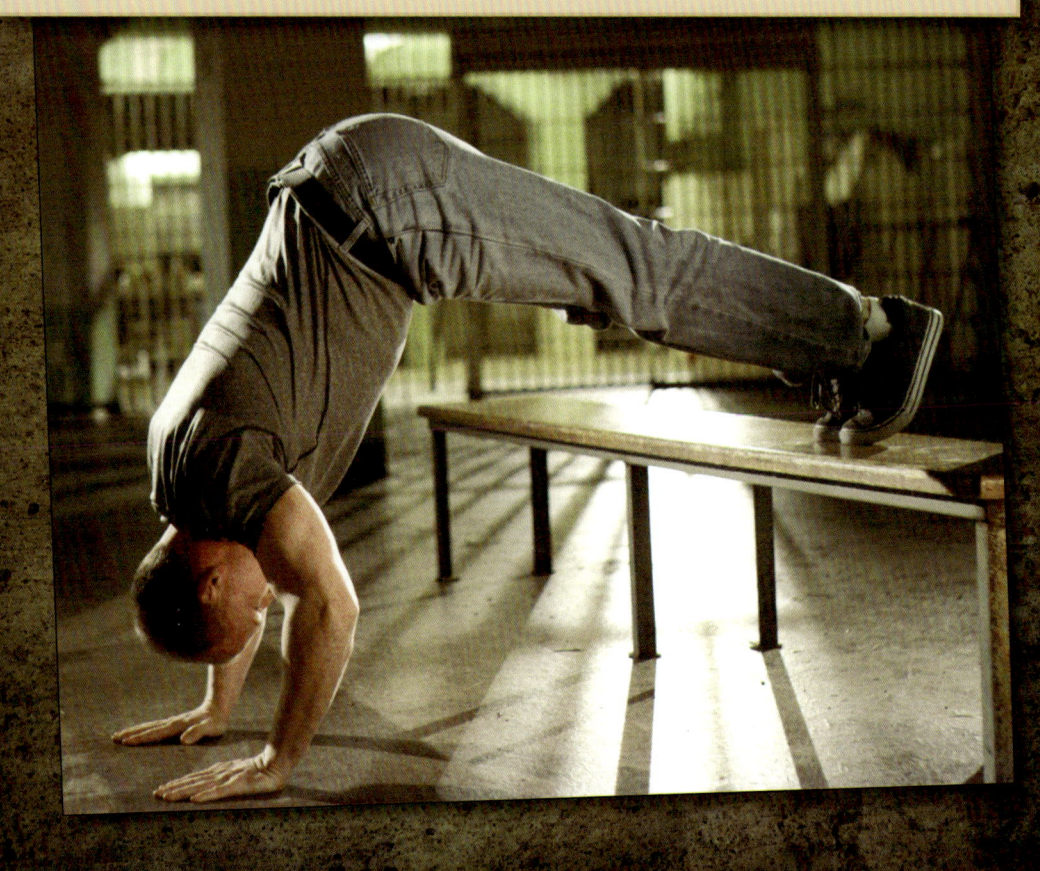

CONVICT CONDITIONING ULTIMATE BODYWEIGHT TRAINING LOG

DAY: _____

DATE: _____

NO.	EXERCISE	SET 1	SET 2	SET 3	SET 4	SET 5

EXTRAS:

COMMENTS:

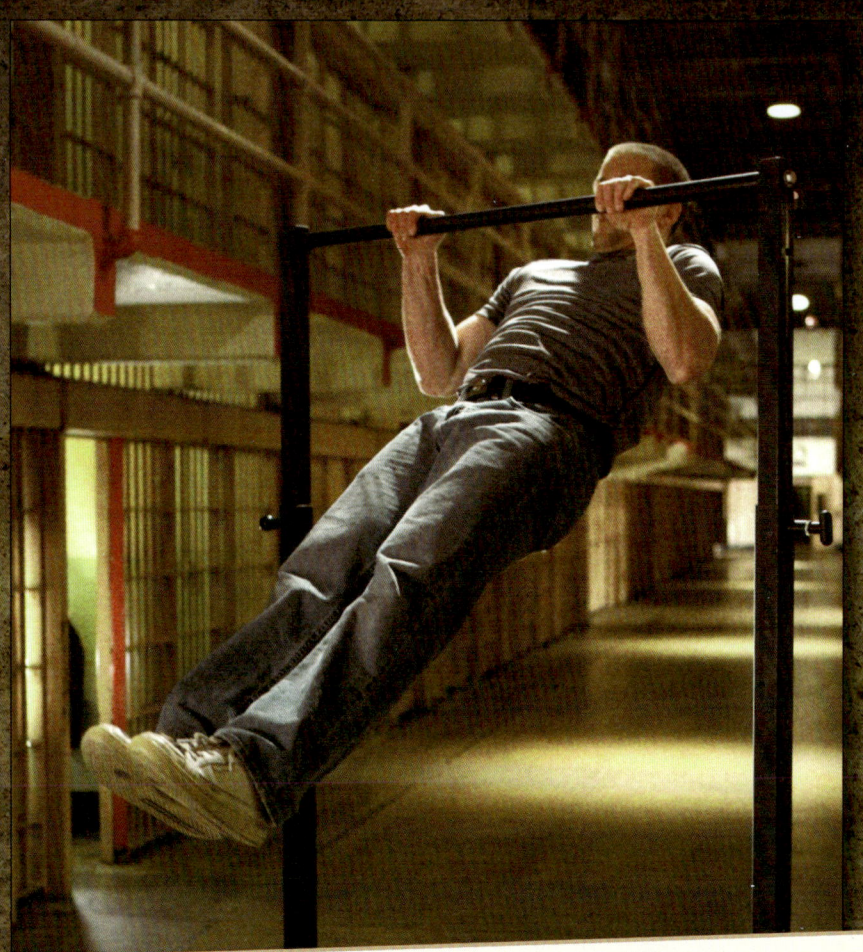

ON ROWS VS PULLUPS:

Many athletes are taught that to work their upper backs, they should bend at the waist and perform bent-over rows. Bending over while holding a heavy weight places huge stresses on the spine and discs—why not go with nature and train with pullups instead? Because your feet aren't in contact with the ground during pullups, the lower back experiences very little stress.

CONVICT CONDITIONING — Ultimate Bodyweight Training Log

DAY: _____
DATE: _____

NO.	EXERCISE	SET 1	SET 2	SET 3	SET 4	SET 5

EXTRAS:

COMMENTS:

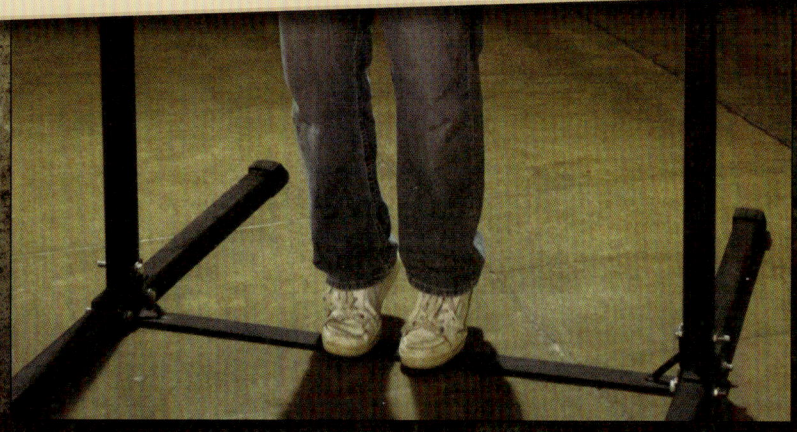

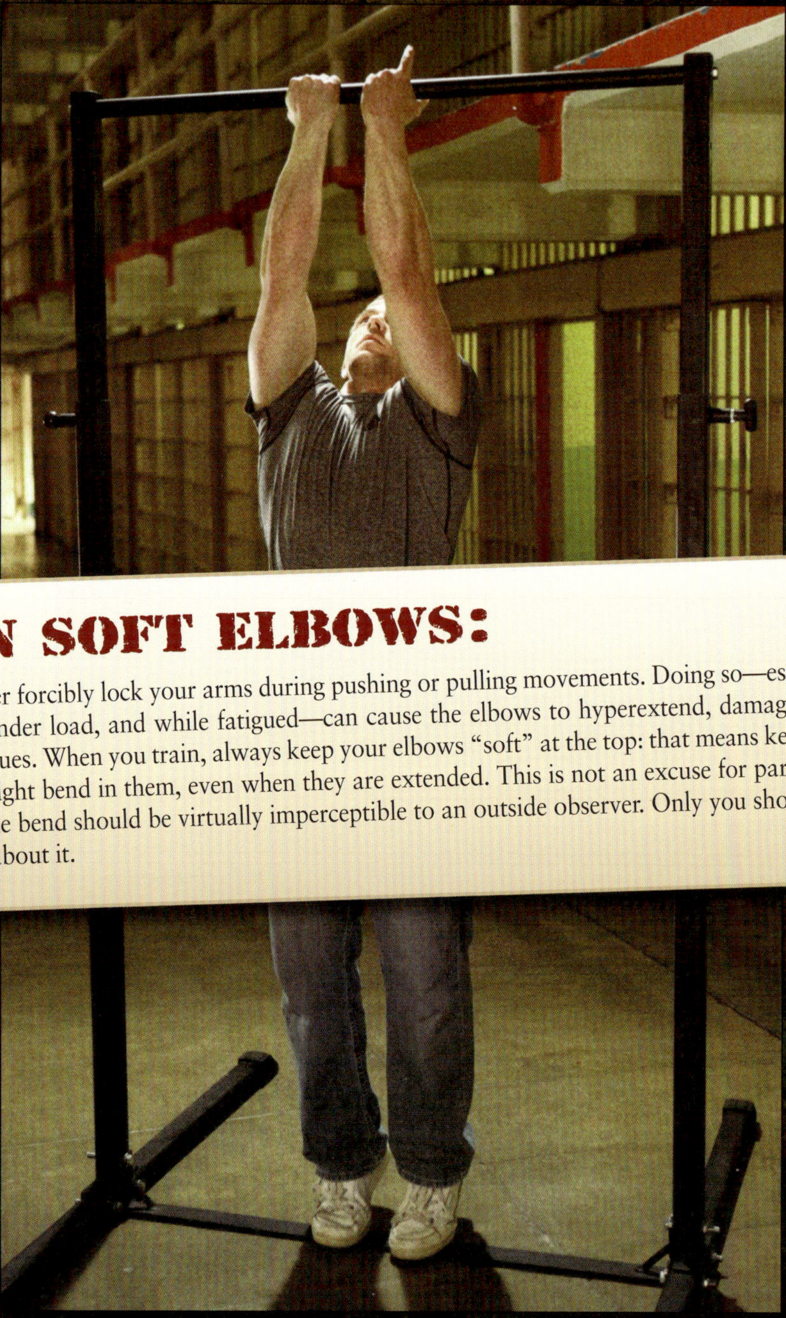

ON SOFT ELBOWS:

Never forcibly lock your arms during pushing or pulling movements. Doing so—especially under load, and while fatigued—can cause the elbows to hyperextend, damaging soft tissues. When you train, always keep your elbows "soft" at the top: that means keeping a slight bend in them, even when they are extended. This is not an excuse for partial reps: the bend should be virtually imperceptible to an outside observer. Only you should know about it.

Paul "Coach" Wade's CONVICT CONDITIONING — Ultimate Bodyweight Training Log

DAY: _____

DATE: _____

NO.	EXERCISE	SET 1	SET 2	SET 3	SET 4	SET 5

EXTRAS:

COMMENTS:

ON TRAINING TO FAILURE:

Many bodybuilders talk about going to "failure" during a hard set; they push themselves until they cannot control their muscles any more. This is a bad plan to apply to calisthenics, because you should be controlling your body at all times—that's the whole idea behind bodyweight training. Avoid "failure" and always keep a rep or two in the bank in order to finish your set safely.

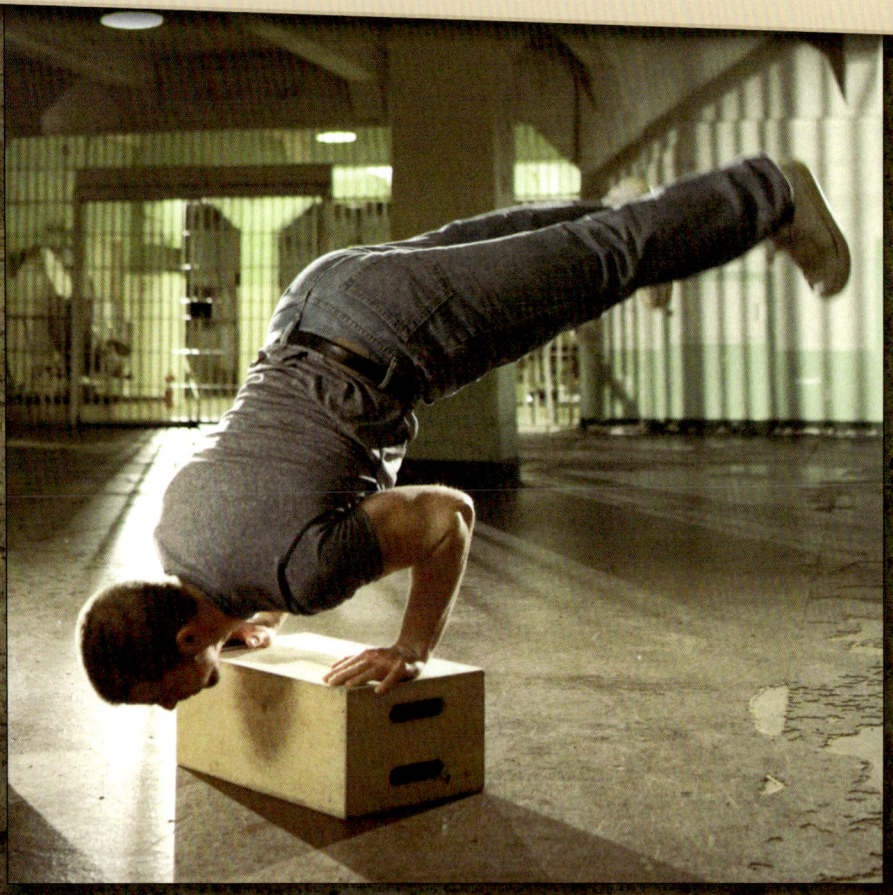

PAUL "COACH" WADE'S CONVICT CONDITIONING ULTIMATE BODYWEIGHT TRAINING LOG

DAY: _____
DATE: _____

NO.	EXERCISE	SET 1	SET 2	SET 3	SET 4	SET 5

EXTRAS:

COMMENTS:

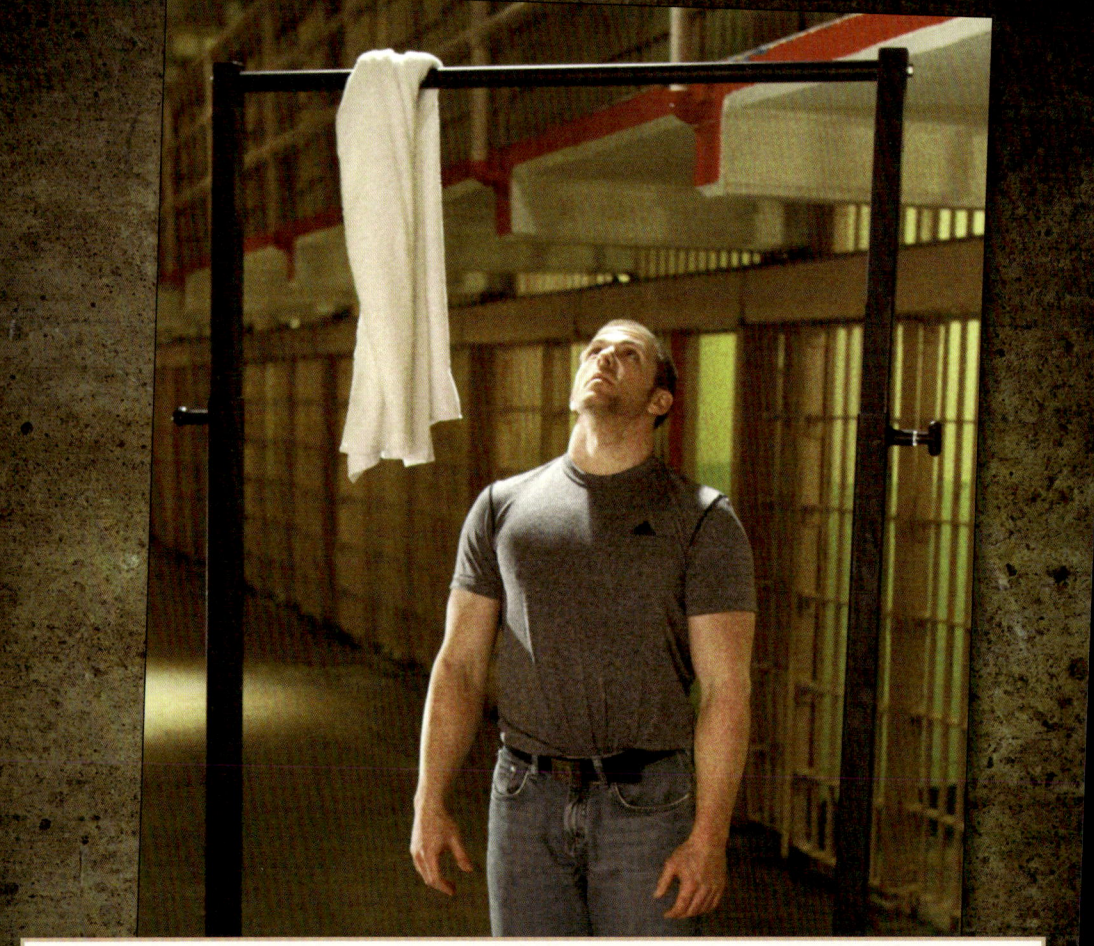

ON TOTAL HAND STRENGTH:

Many gym-trained athletes have surprisingly underdeveloped hand strength. They may have strong *fingers*—from holding a barbell or dumbbells—but rarely do they have powerful *thumbs*, and this is what limits their total hand power. Military men rarely have this weakness, because they are forced to climb ropes. The thumbs can be strengthened to a high level by performing hangs or pullups gripping a towel or two slung around the overhead bar.

PAUL "COACH" WADE'S CONVICT CONDITIONING — Ultimate Bodyweight Training Log

117

DAY: _____

DATE: _____

NO.	EXERCISE	SET 1	SET 2	SET 3	SET 4	SET 5

EXTRAS:

COMMENTS:

On Range-of-Motion:

To keep your joints and tendons strong and healthy, you should always be using full-range movements in your training: full-range squats, pullups and pushups especially. Sometimes during your progress you need to explore partial movements to gradually work into harder techniques, but when you apply short-range movements, these should *always* be complemented by easier full-range techniques somewhere in your workout.

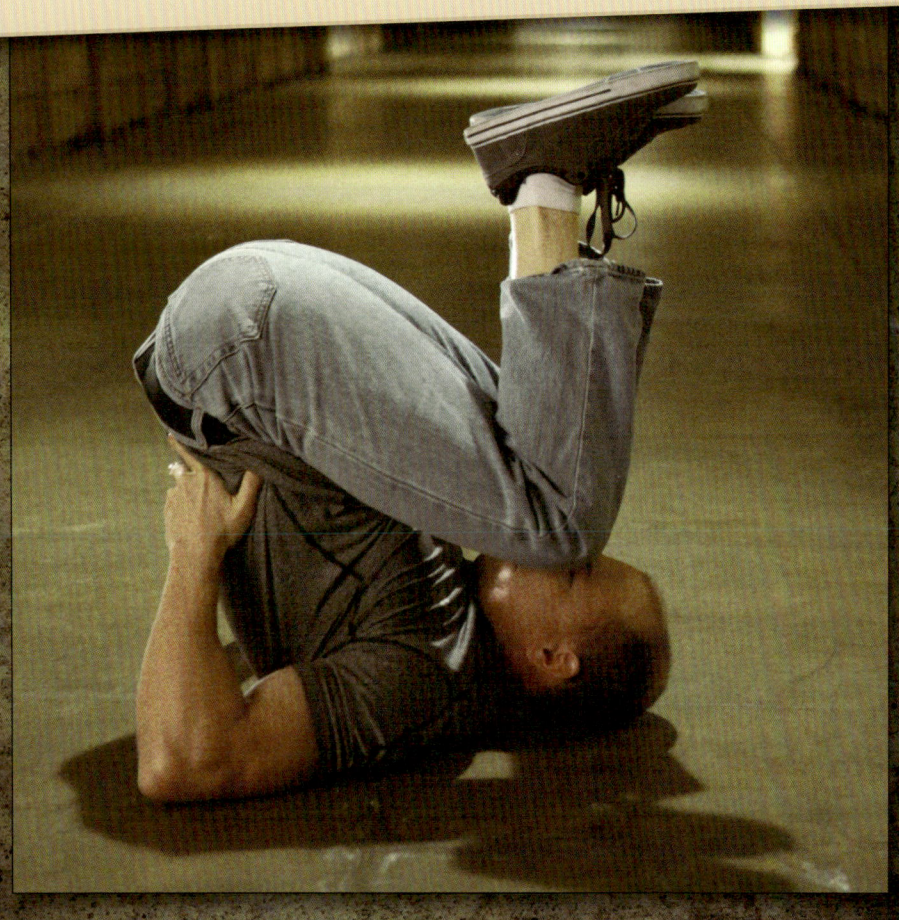

CONVICT CONDITIONING ULTIMATE BODYWEIGHT TRAINING LOG

DAY: _____
DATE: _____

NO.	EXERCISE	SET 1	SET 2	SET 3	SET 4	SET 5

EXTRAS:

COMMENTS:

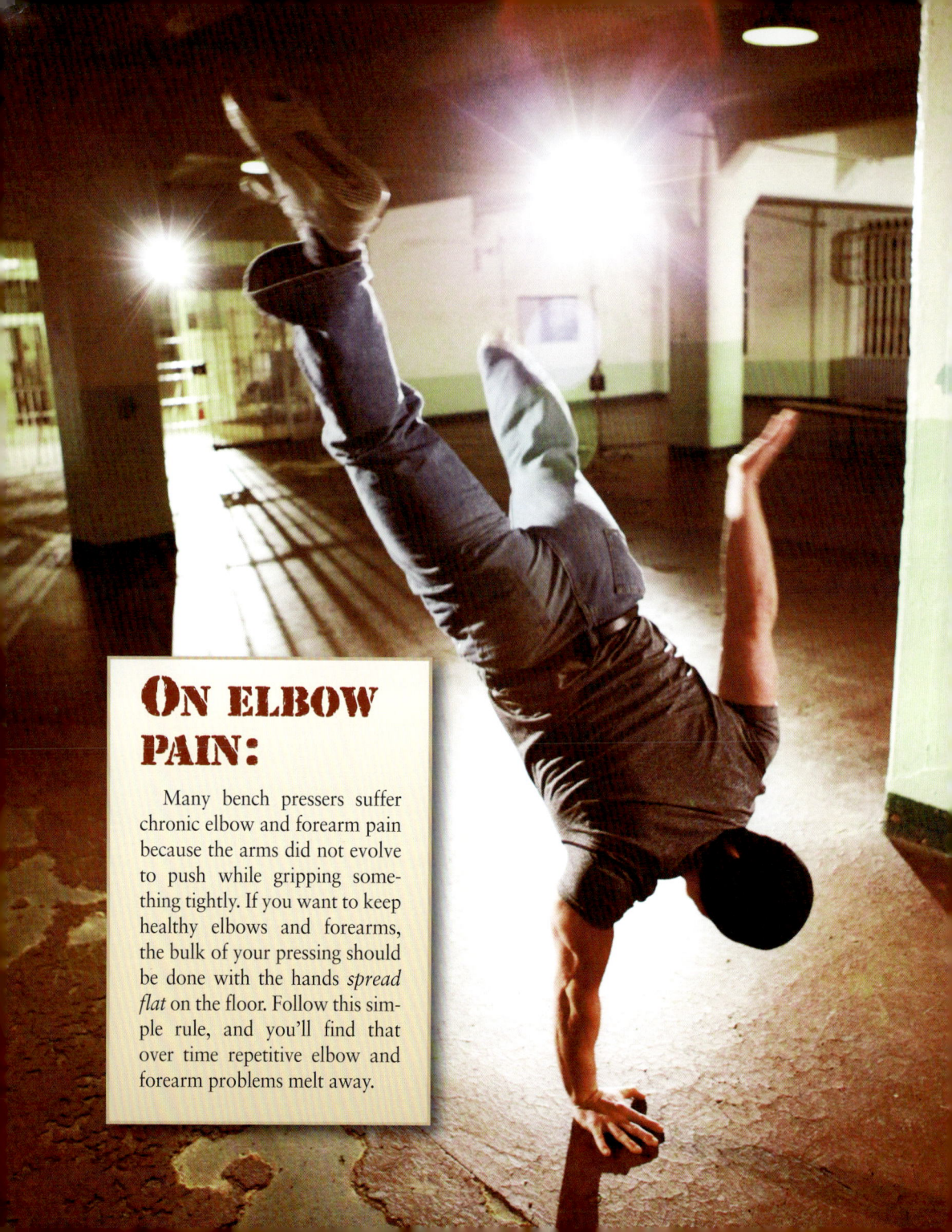

ON ELBOW PAIN:

Many bench pressers suffer chronic elbow and forearm pain because the arms did not evolve to push while gripping something tightly. If you want to keep healthy elbows and forearms, the bulk of your pressing should be done with the hands *spread flat* on the floor. Follow this simple rule, and you'll find that over time repetitive elbow and forearm problems melt away.

CONVICT CONDITIONING — Ultimate Bodyweight Training Log

DAY: _____

DATE: _____

NO.	EXERCISE	SET 1	SET 2	SET 3	SET 4	SET 5

EXTRAS:

COMMENTS:

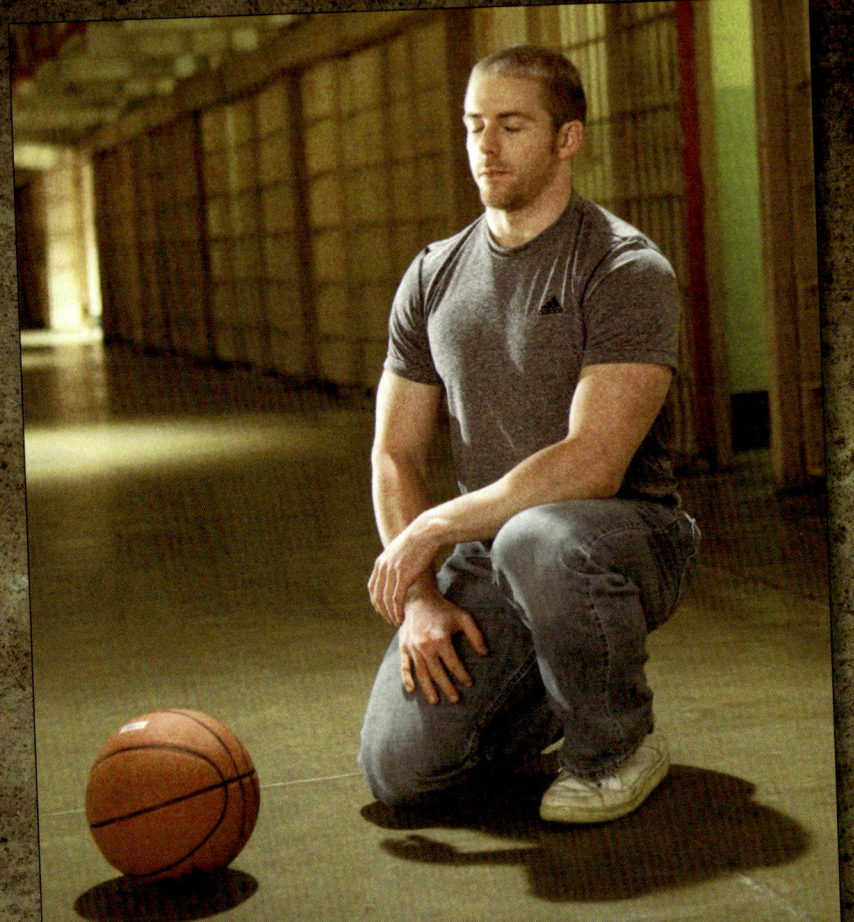

On rest between sets:

One mistake beginners in old school calisthenics often make is rushing from set to set. Powerlifters understand that to gain added mass and power, you need to take a little extra rest after each set, to gear up for the next effort. Bodyweight strength work is no different. Rest as long as you need to between sets, but try not to exceed five minutes—or your muscles will get cold.

CONVICT CONDITIONING ULTIMATE BODYWEIGHT TRAINING LOG

DAY: _____
DATE: _____

NO.	EXERCISE	SET 1	SET 2	SET 3	SET 4	SET 5

EXTRAS:

COMMENTS:

ONE-LEG SQUAT RECORD:

Who says a leg workout needs to take hours? In 2012 Silvio Sabba performed 50 one-leg squats in just under a minute. Throw in a minute's rest, and for both legs that's only a three minute workout. Any takers?

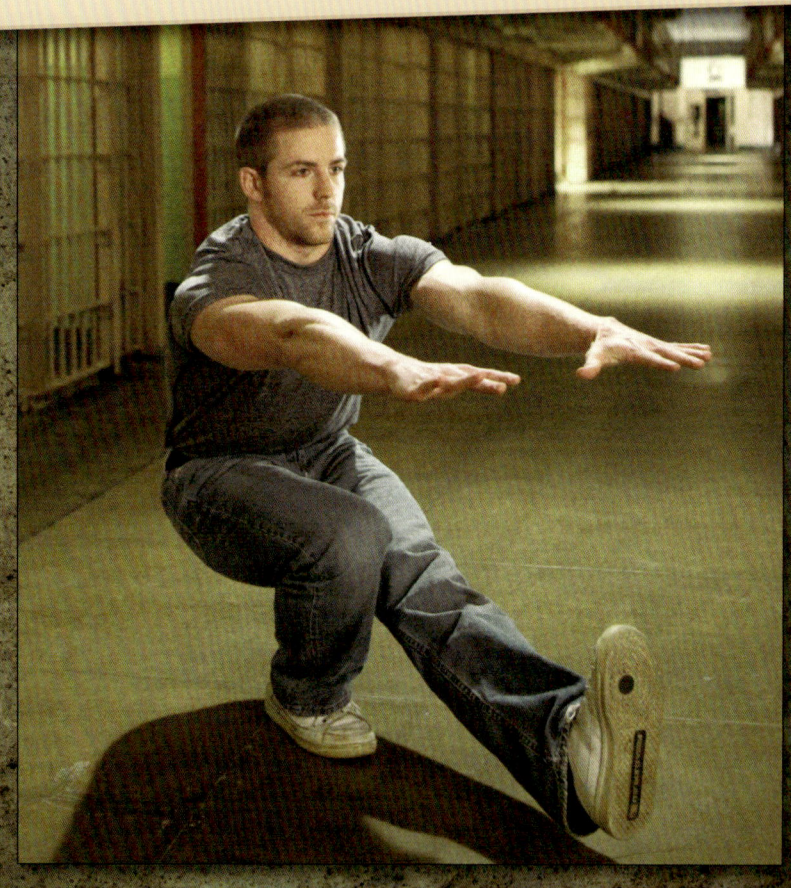

PAUL "COACH" WADE'S CONVICT CONDITIONING
ULTIMATE BODYWEIGHT TRAINING LOG

DAY: _____

DATE: _____

NO.	EXERCISE	SET 1	SET 2	SET 3	SET 4	SET 5

EXTRAS:

COMMENTS:

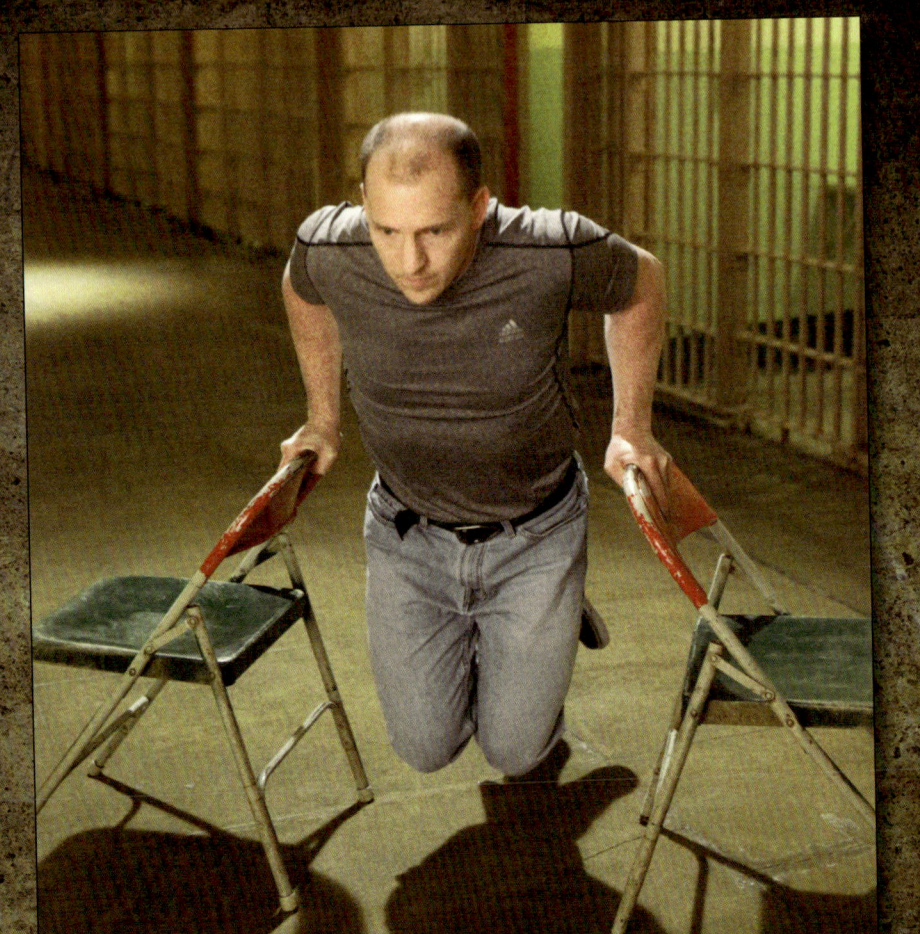

On dips:

Dips between chairs or on the parallel bars are a good exercise, provided you can do them without incurring joint pain: some athletes just can't do dips without hurting their shoulders or sternum. One of the problems with dips is that once you can do them fairly well, it's difficult to make them progressive. This is why most convict-athletes stick with prison pushups, which can be taken to an almost impossible level of difficulty.

PAUL "COACH" WADE'S CONVICT CONDITIONING
Ultimate Bodyweight Training Log

DAY:_____
DATE:_____

NO.	EXERCISE	SET 1	SET 2	SET 3	SET 4	SET 5

EXTRAS:

COMMENTS:

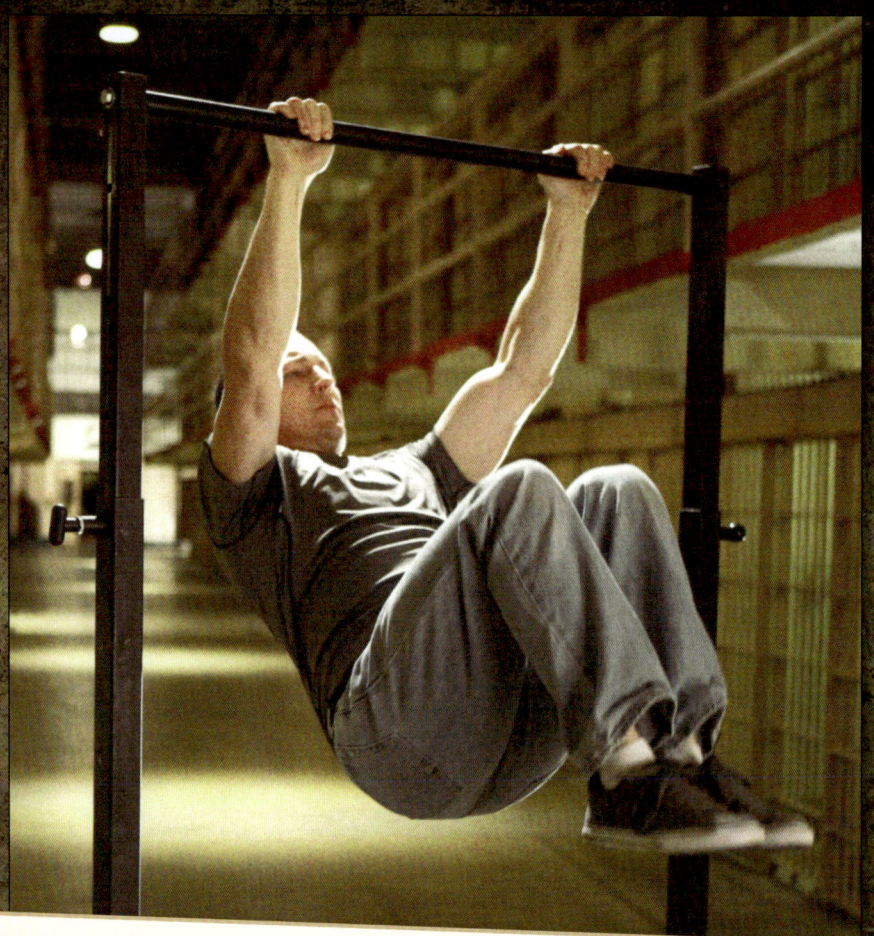

ON SPOT REDUCTION:

The idea that you can burn fat from a specific area of your body by working that area—also known as *spot reduction*—has been proven to be a myth. But that doesn't mean that you shouldn't train those out-of-shape areas! Training a flabby body part will increase blood flow in the region, tone up loose muscles and tighten up the skin (which is attached to muscle tissue). If in doubt…work it out!

Paul "Coach" Wade's CONVICT CONDITIONING Ultimate Bodyweight Training Log

DAY: _____

DATE: _____

NO.	EXERCISE	SET 1	SET 2	SET 3	SET 4	SET 5

EXTRAS:

COMMENTS:

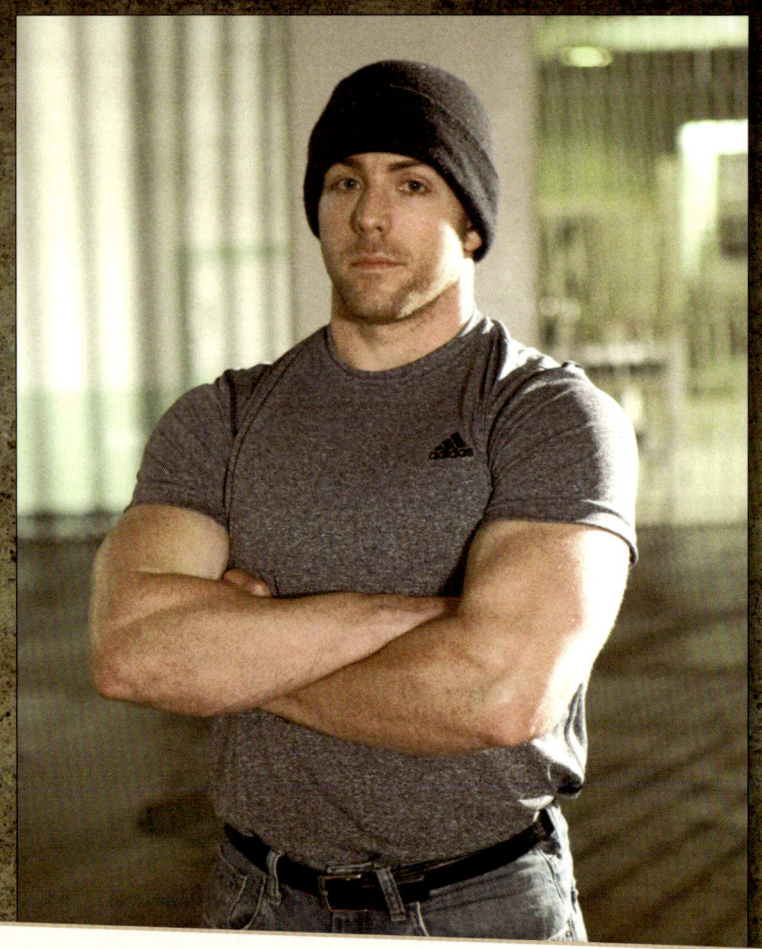

ON UPPER BODY SIZE:

The idea that you need heavy bars and other weights to build a muscular upper body is a commonly held myth. Look at Olympic gymnasts and you'll see that many of them possess truly *huge* upper bodies—achieved without touching a single weight! When you see bodybuilders bigger than calisthenics masters, this is not because those bodybuilders are using superior training methods: it's because they are using anabolic steroids and other tissue-building drugs.

PAUL "COACH" WADE'S CONVICT CONDITIONING — Ultimate Bodyweight Training Log

DAY: _____

DATE: _____

NO.	EXERCISE	SET 1	SET 2	SET 3	SET 4	SET 5

EXTRAS:

COMMENTS:

ON NON-STOP PUSHUPS:

What's your idea of a high rep set of pushups? 50 reps? A hundred? These ideas are just numbers, and the trained body is capable of much, much more. In 1980, Japan's Minoru Yoshida performed 10,507 pushups...non-stop.

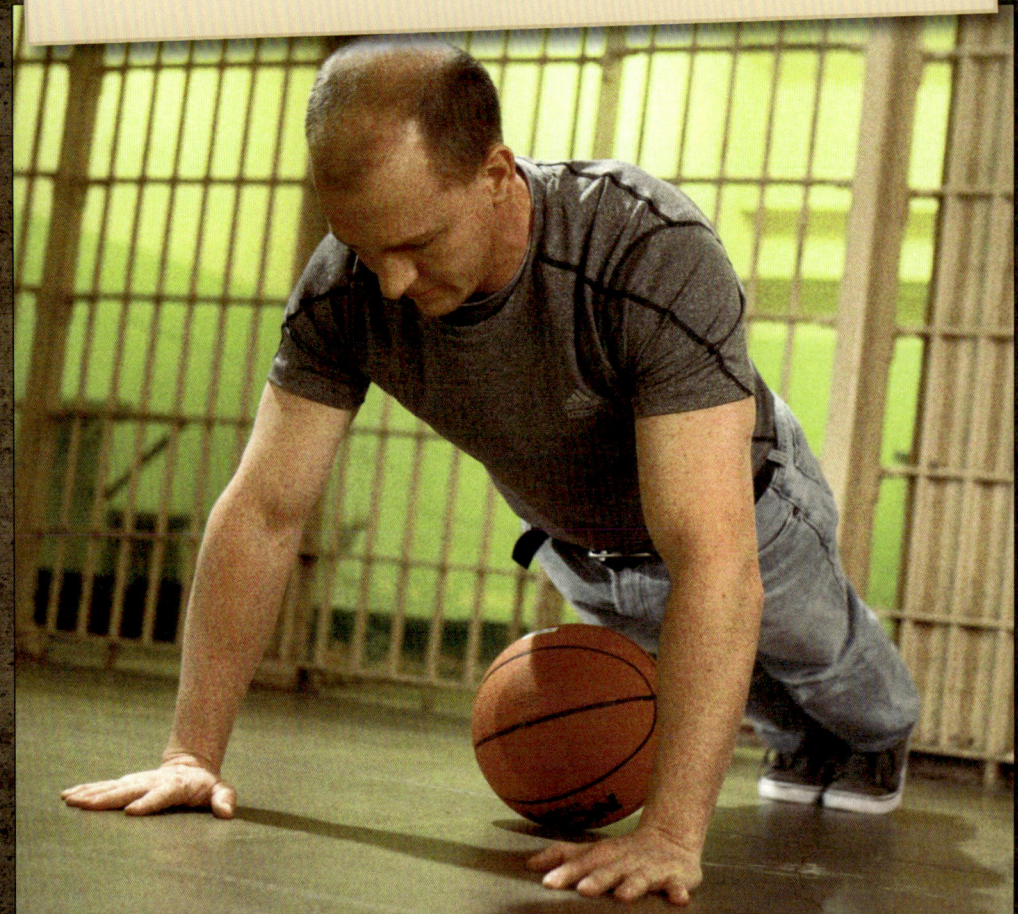

PAUL "COACH" WADE'S CONVICT CONDITIONING — Ultimate Bodyweight Training Log

DAY: _____

DATE: _____

NO.	EXERCISE	SET 1	SET 2	SET 3	SET 4	SET 5

EXTRAS:

COMMENTS:

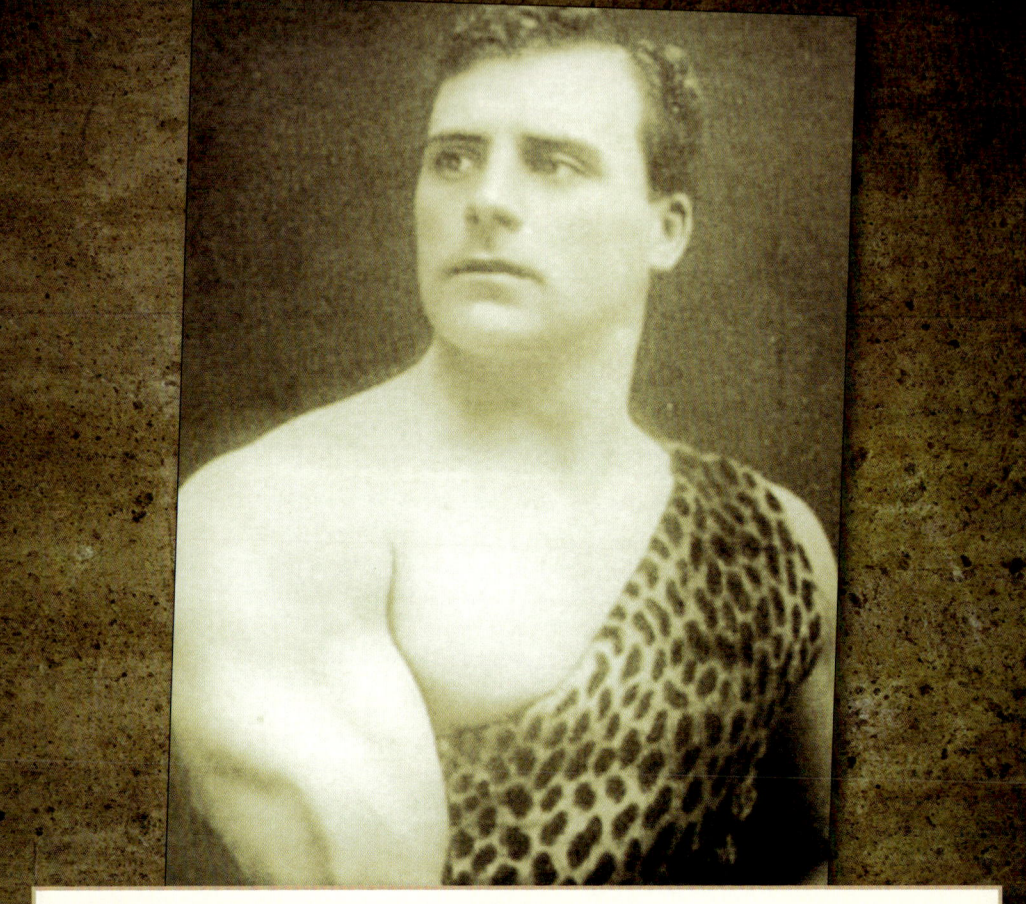

ON ROPE CLIMBING:

Climbing a rope makes for a phenomenal bodyweight workout. Supporting yourself on a vertical rope is harder than hanging from a horizontal bar, so rope work gives you stronger hands. A strong grip makes for a strong arm, and rope climbers can be easily identified by their huge biceps: the biggest muscular arms in the pre-steroid era belonged to William Bankier, a Scotsman whose only bicep exercise was rope climbing.

PAUL "COACH" WADE'S CONVICT CONDITIONING — Ultimate Bodyweight Training Log

DAY: _____

DATE: _____

NO.	EXERCISE	SET 1	SET 2	SET 3	SET 4	SET 5

EXTRAS:

COMMENTS:

On "Bodypart Training":

The body evolved to work as a unit, so don't isolate your muscles when you workout. When you train, don't think in terms of *body parts*—for example, don't think "I'm gonna train pecs today", or "Wednesday is lats day". Instead, learn to think in terms of *exercises*: think "I'm gonna do some pushups" or "today I'll beat my pullup record". Ironically, this is the best way to bulk up all your individual muscles.

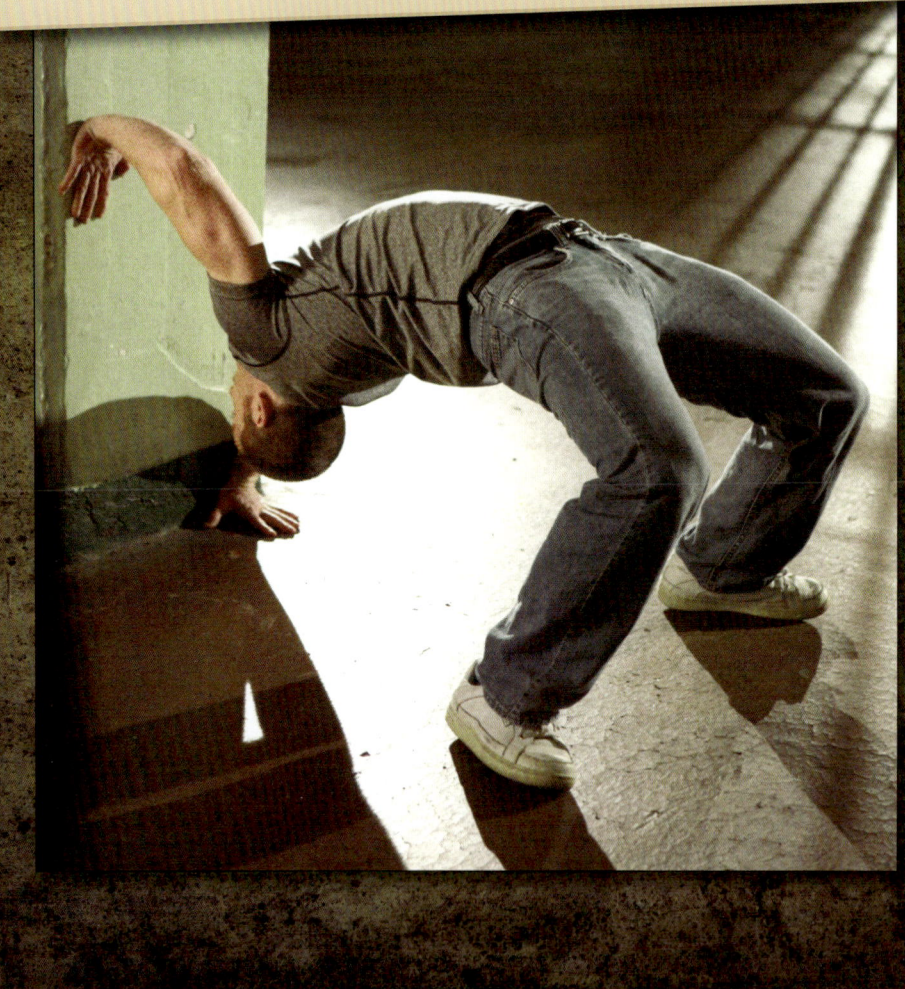

PAUL "COACH" WADE'S CONVICT CONDITIONING
ULTIMATE BODYWEIGHT TRAINING LOG

DAY: _____
DATE: _____

NO.	EXERCISE	SET 1	SET 2	SET 3	SET 4	SET 5

EXTRAS:

COMMENTS:

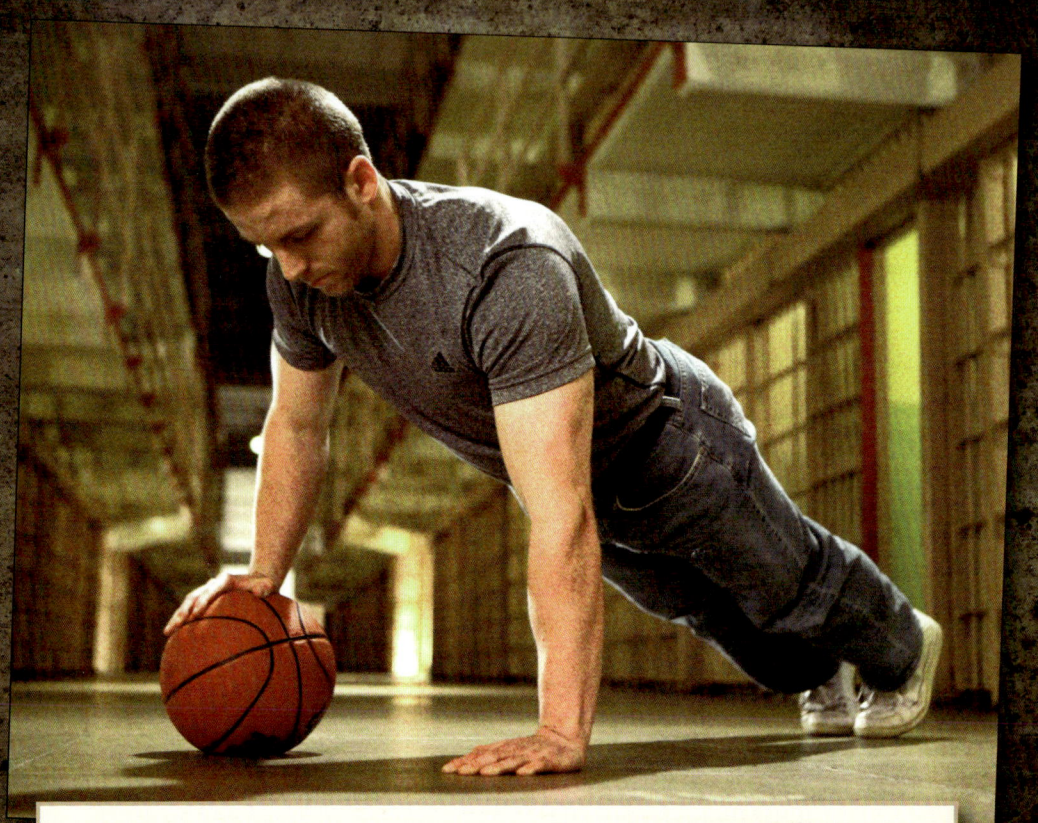

ON BASKETBALL WORK:

One of the finest pieces of training equipment for the bodyweight athlete is a humble basketball. Doing your pushups with one hand on a ball forces you to build stabilization strength deep in the shoulders, and this effectively bulletproofs the rotator cuff and other internal tissues. Forget expensive training gadgets: find a good quality, tacky-gripped ball, and it will last you for years.

PAUL "COACH" WADE'S CONVICT CONDITIONING
ULTIMATE BODYWEIGHT TRAINING LOG

DAY: _____
DATE: _____

NO.	EXERCISE	SET 1	SET 2	SET 3	SET 4	SET 5

EXTRAS:

COMMENTS:

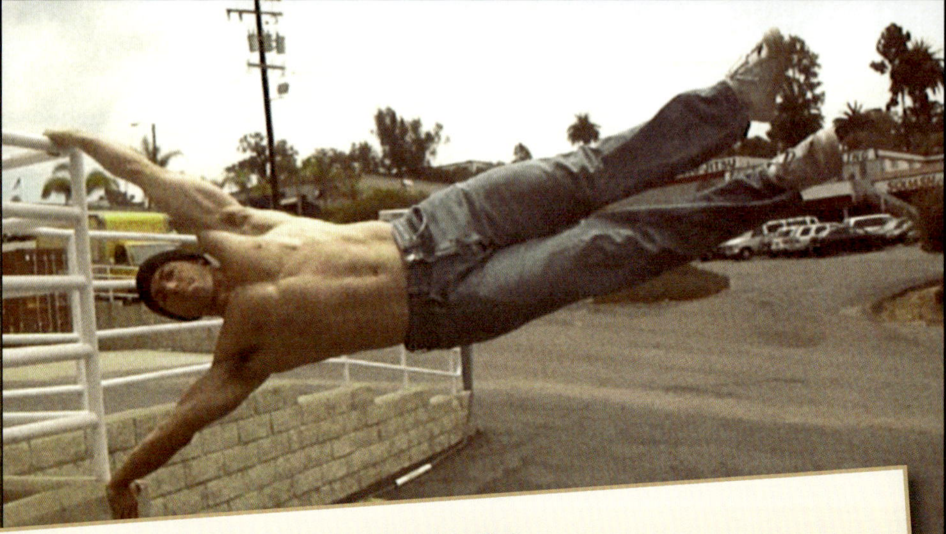

On the Flanks:

It is impossible to achieve great strength or athleticism if you neglect what strongmen used to call the *flanks*—the muscles running up the side of the body. The most efficient (and safest) way to work these muscles is with the flag family of movements. Flags work every muscle in the side of the body, from side-thigh to hips and obliques, plus serratus and lats! A complete progressive course of flag exercises is contained in *Convict Conditioning 2.*

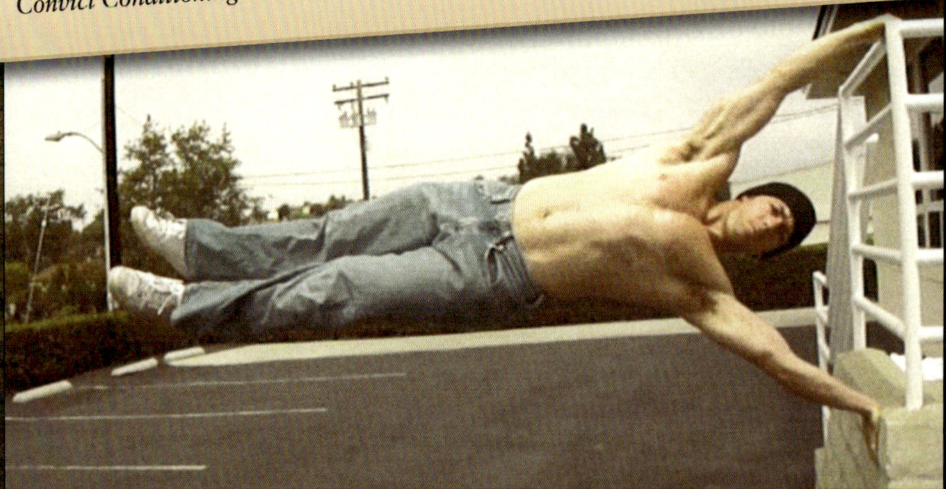

PAUL "COACH" WADE'S CONVICT CONDITIONING ULTIMATE BODYWEIGHT TRAINING LOG

DAY: _____
DATE: _____

NO.	EXERCISE	SET 1	SET 2	SET 3	SET 4	SET 5

EXTRAS:

COMMENTS:

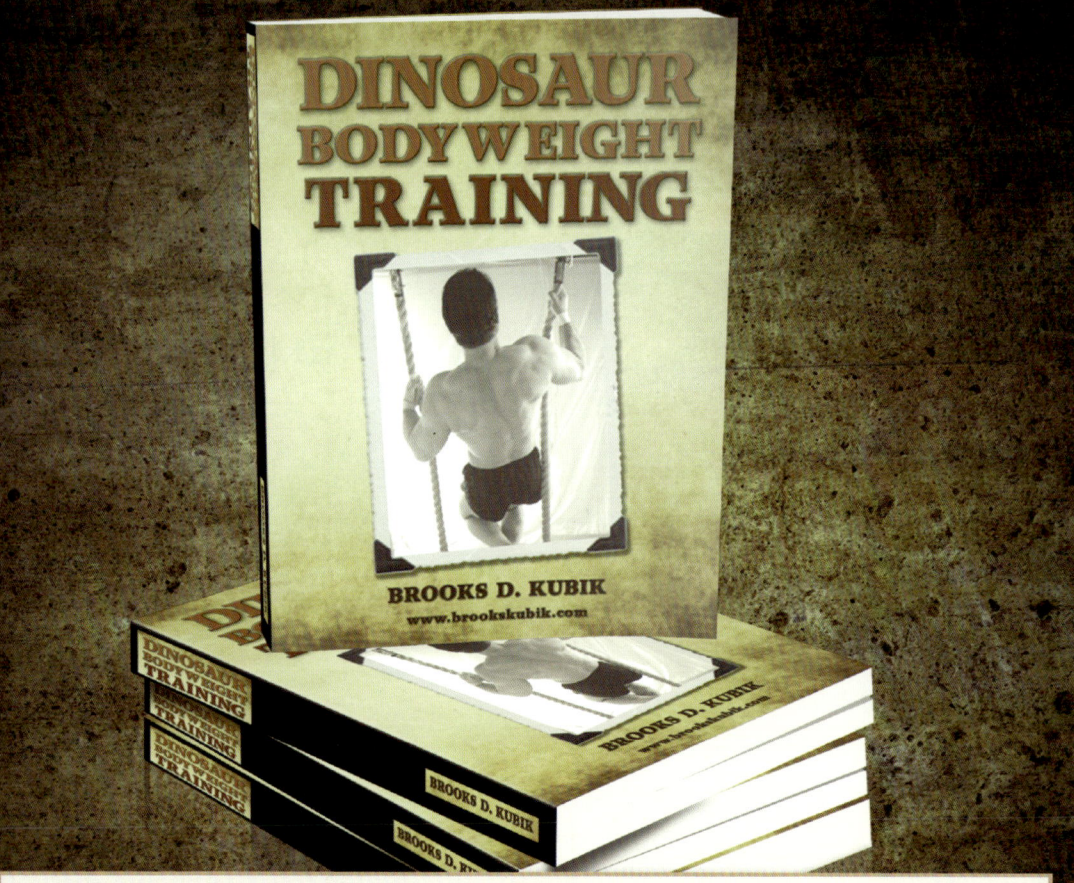

Great Bodyweight Strength Books # 4: Dinosaur Bodyweight Training —Brooks Kubik

This is a unique (and often surprising) look at strength calisthenics from one of the world's most famous iron lifters. After decades of pushing and pulling bone-crushing weights, Brook's shoulders were crunching like broken glass. He dropped the weights and developed his own brutal system of bodyweight training. He not only retained his phenomenal strength, he also built slabs of new muscle, and healed his body to the degree that he was soon hitting the super-heavy weights again.

PAUL "COACH" WADE'S CONVICT CONDITIONING ULTIMATE BODYWEIGHT TRAINING LOG

143

DAY: _____
DATE: _____

NO.	EXERCISE	SET 1	SET 2	SET 3	SET 4	SET 5

EXTRAS:

COMMENTS:

ON EQUIPMENT:

Most of the workout equipment on the market today is designed to make your training *easier*—which is the opposite of what you want if you are going to fulfill your potential. As a general rule of thumb, the more complex a workout tool or gadget is, the more useless it is. Over time train yourself to get by with *less and less* equipment—not *more*. Make your body your gymnasium, and it will reward you.

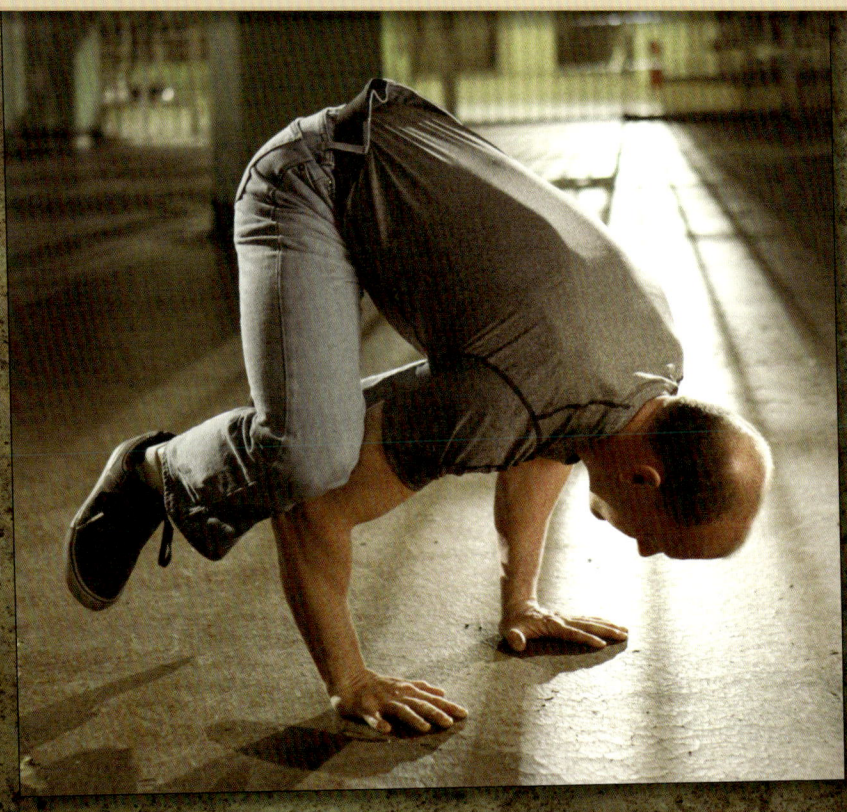

CONVICT CONDITIONING — Ultimate Bodyweight Training Log

DAY: _____

DATE: _____

NO.	EXERCISE	SET 1	SET 2	SET 3	SET 4	SET 5

EXTRAS:

COMMENTS:

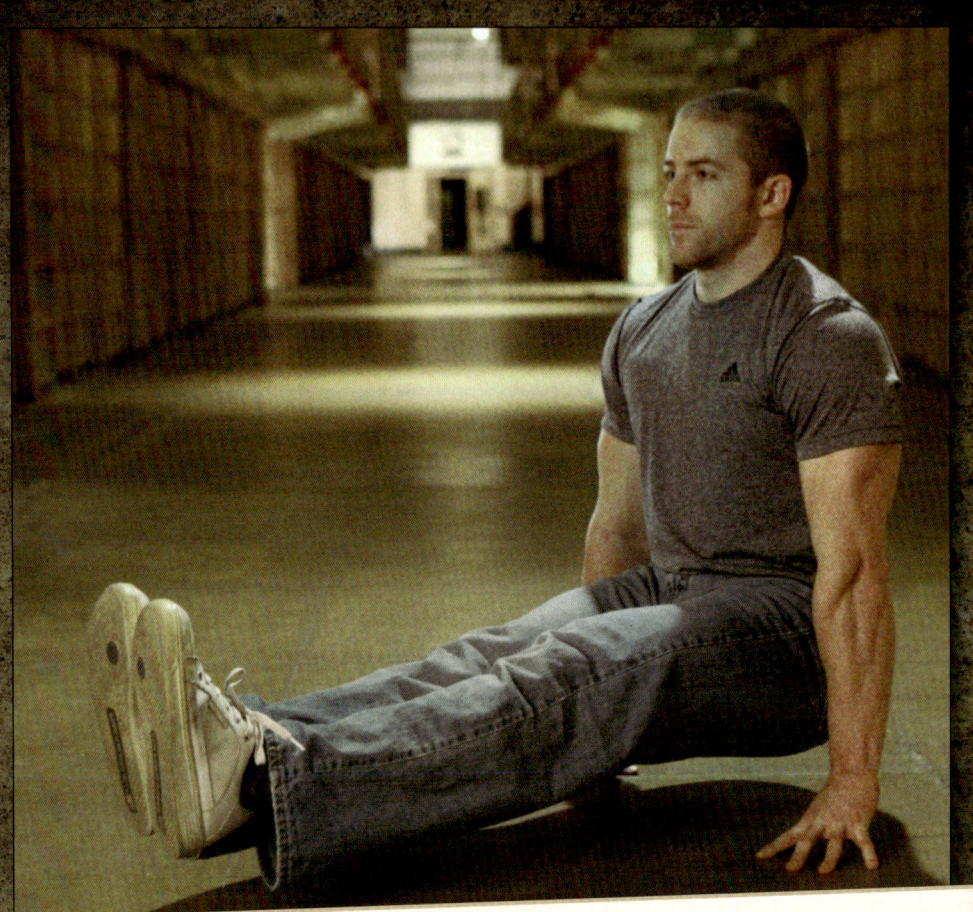

ON PROGRESSIVE CLIMBING:

Like any other calisthenics activity, rope climbing can be made progressive. At first, try to get up and down a rope using your hands and feet. Once this gets easier, begin going down using only your hands. Before long, you'll be going up using only arm power—no legs. Many elite rope climbers begin the rope climb seated on the floor, and continue climbing with their legs in the L-hold position to ensure zero lower body help.

PAUL "COACH" WADE'S CONVICT CONDITIONING
Ultimate Bodyweight Training Log

DAY: _____

DATE: _____

NO.	EXERCISE	SET 1	SET 2	SET 3	SET 4	SET 5

EXTRAS:

COMMENTS:

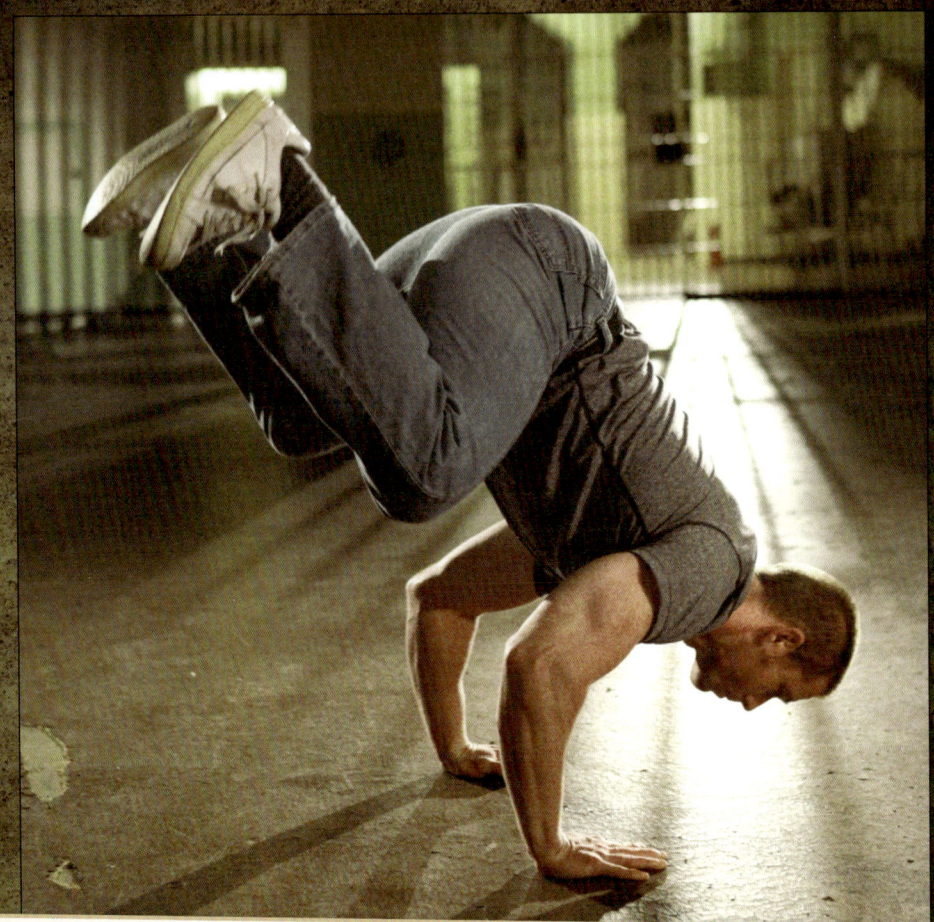

ON NUTRITION:

When it comes to nutrition, I like to keep things simple. The question; *am I eating enough?* can be answered by asking; *am I consistently making progress in my training?* If the answer is "yes", then you are eating enough. If you are putting on weight week after week, then you are eating too damn much. Simple, huh?

PAUL "COACH" WADE'S CONVICT CONDITIONING ULTIMATE BODYWEIGHT TRAINING LOG

149

DAY: _____
DATE: _____

NO.	EXERCISE	SET 1	SET 2	SET 3	SET 4	SET 5

EXTRAS:

COMMENTS:

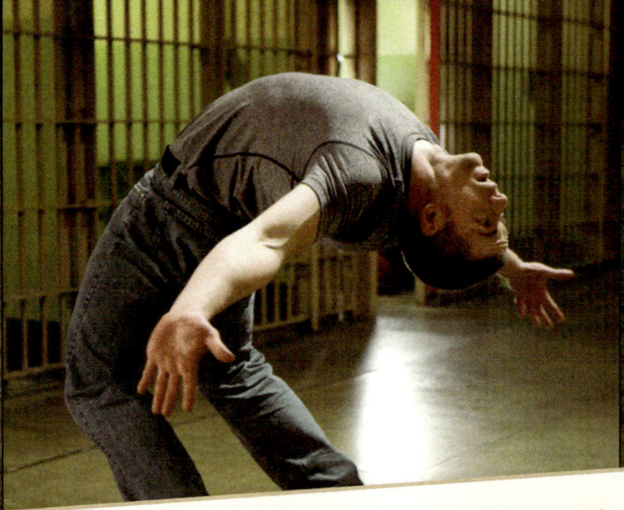

ON A COMPLETE BACK:

For a fully developed back, it's a good idea to perform at least three exercises regularly: a *vertical pull* for the lats, a *horizontal pull* for the upper back, and a *spinal exercise*. For a vertical pull, choose from the pullup family of movements; for a horizontal pull try horizontal pullups of different types, or front levers on a bar. For spinal work, nothing beats bridges, baby!

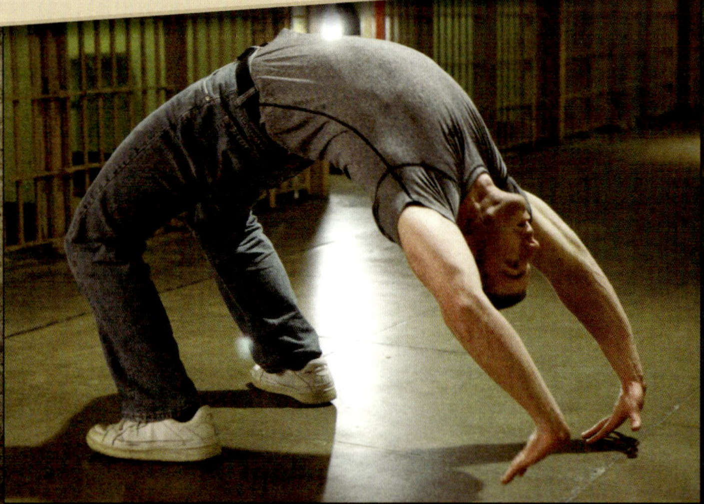

CONVICT CONDITIONING ULTIMATE BODYWEIGHT TRAINING LOG

DAY: _____
DATE: _____

NO.	EXERCISE	SET 1	SET 2	SET 3	SET 4	SET 5

EXTRAS:

COMMENTS:

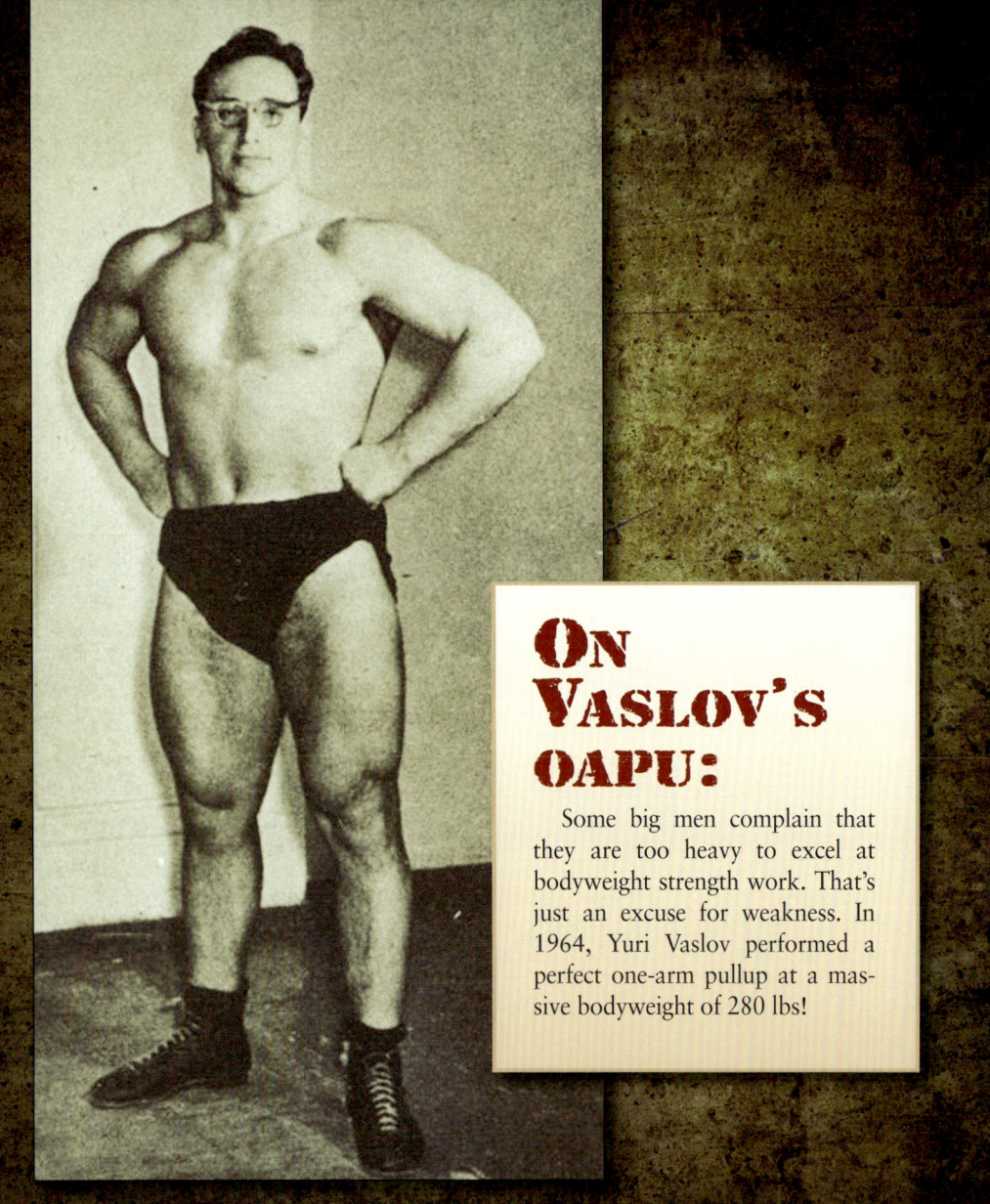

On Vaslov's OAPU:

Some big men complain that they are too heavy to excel at bodyweight strength work. That's just an excuse for weakness. In 1964, Yuri Vaslov performed a perfect one-arm pullup at a massive bodyweight of 280 lbs!

CONVICT CONDITIONING — Ultimate Bodyweight TRAINING LOG

DAY: _____
DATE: _____

NO.	EXERCISE	SET 1	SET 2	SET 3	SET 4	SET 5

EXTRAS:

COMMENTS:

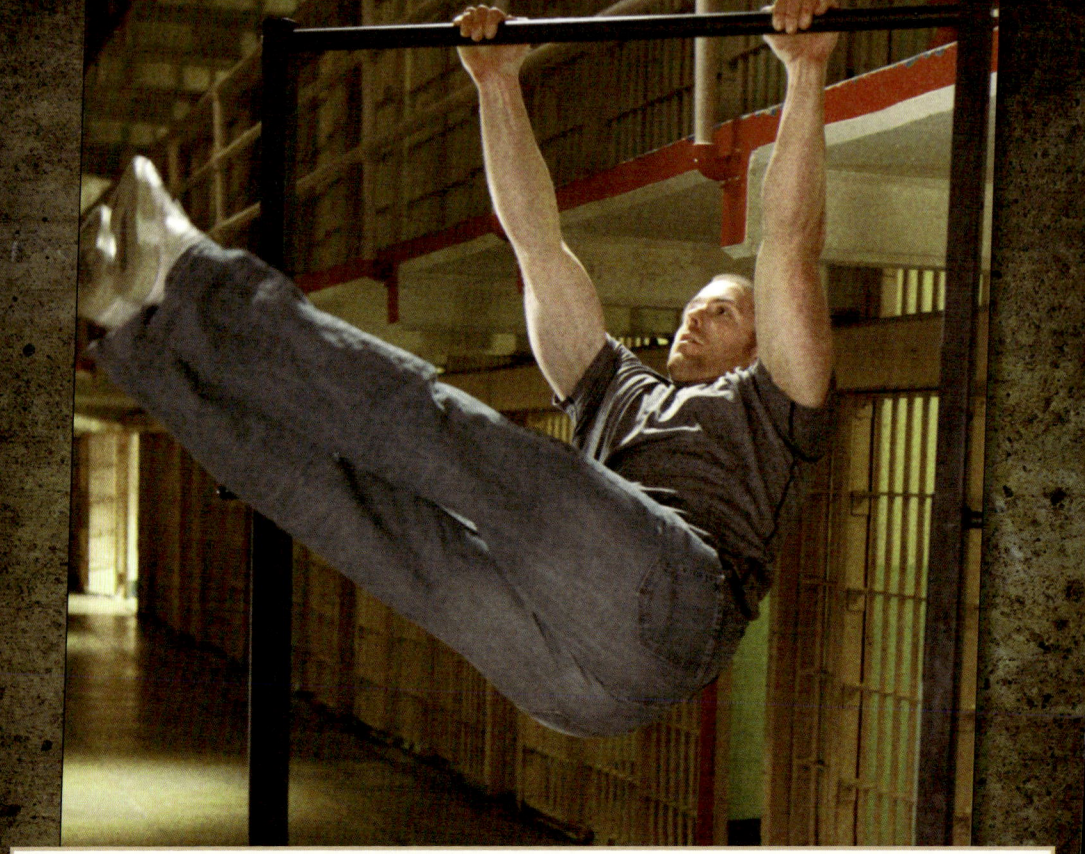

ON THE SUBCONSCIOUS EFFECT:

I very rarely train a student in old school calisthenics who doesn't noticeably drop body fat—even if they're not trying. This can be explained by what I call the *subconscious effect*. If you are busting your butt to increase reps on tough exercises like pushups, pullups and squats, your primitive brain-stem realizes that it's struggling to move the body and jettisons some of the excess flab. Try calisthenics for three months and watch this happen.

PAUL "COACH" WADE'S CONVICT CONDITIONING ULTIMATE BODYWEIGHT TRAINING LOG

DAY: _____

DATE: _____

NO.	EXERCISE	SET 1	SET 2	SET 3	SET 4	SET 5

EXTRAS:

COMMENTS:

On Bob Jones:

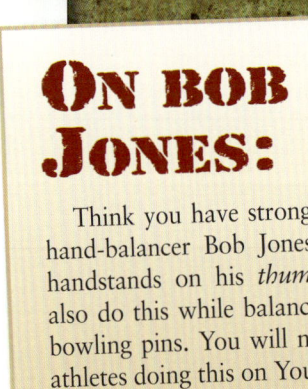

Think you have strong hands? The great hand-balancer Bob Jones used to perform handstands on his *thumbs*—and he could also do this while balancing on a couple of bowling pins. You will not see any modern athletes doing this on Youtube.

CONVICT CONDITIONING — ULTIMATE BODYWEIGHT TRAINING LOG

DAY: _____
DATE: _____

NO.	EXERCISE	SET 1	SET 2	SET 3	SET 4	SET 5

EXTRAS:

COMMENTS:

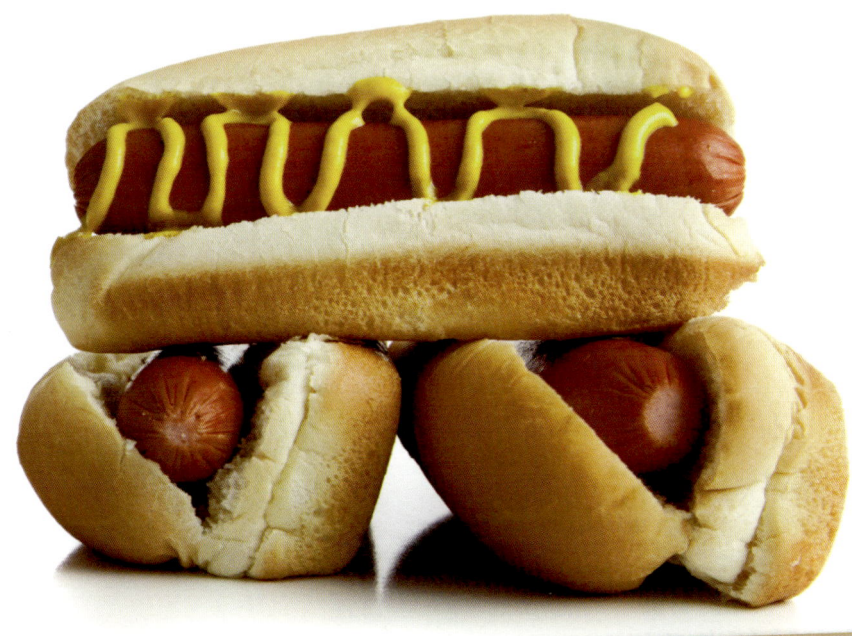

ON HOTDOGS:

On Independence Day 2009, California boy Joseph "Joey" Chestnut consumed an incredible 68 hotdogs, with buns, in just ten minutes. The feat was recorded under official conditions as part of *Nathan's Hot Dog Eating Contest* held yearly in Coney Island. What does this have to do with bodyweight training? Nothing—I'm just seeing if you're paying attention. And I'm hungry.

PAUL "COACH" WADE'S CONVICT CONDITIONING
Ultimate Bodyweight Training Log

159

DAY: _____
DATE: _____

NO.	EXERCISE	SET 1	SET 2	SET 3	SET 4	SET 5

EXTRAS:

COMMENTS:

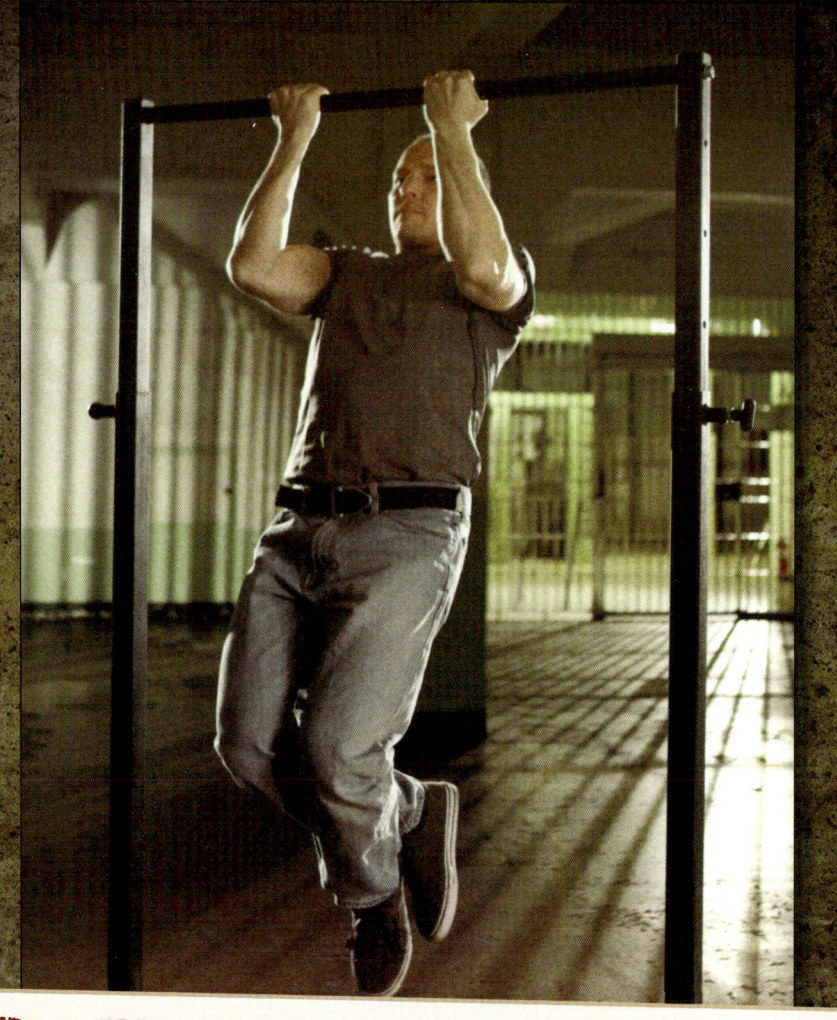

ON YONG'S PULLUPS:

On December 29th 1994, Lee Chin Yong of Korea performed 612 consecutive pullups—the longest nonstop set ever recorded under official conditions. He was 70 years old at the time: a senior citizen. What's your excuse, kid?

CONVICT CONDITIONING — ULTIMATE BODYWEIGHT TRAINING LOG

DAY: _____

DATE: _____

NO.	EXERCISE	SET 1	SET 2	SET 3	SET 4	SET 5

EXTRAS:

COMMENTS:

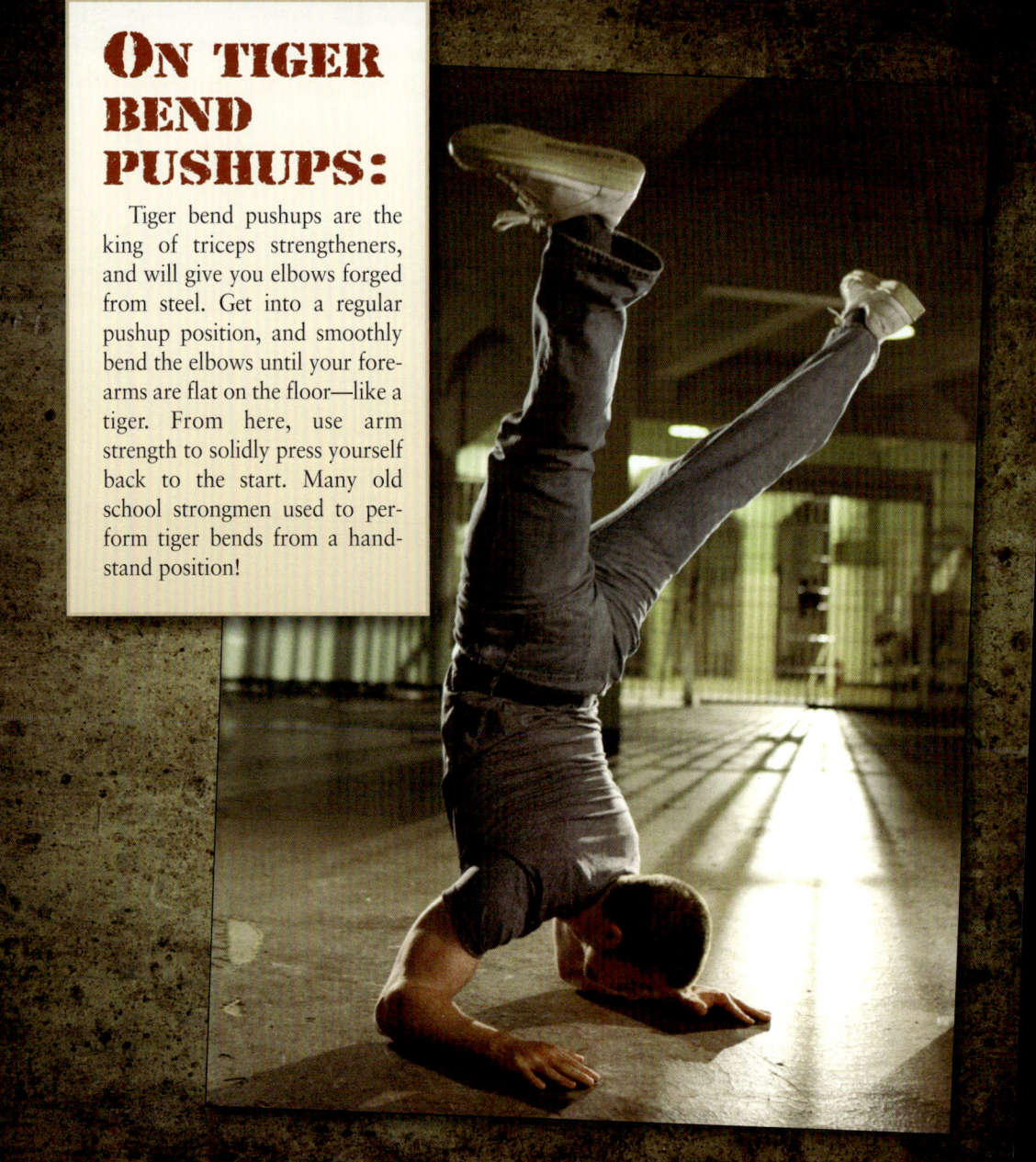

On Tiger Bend Pushups:

Tiger bend pushups are the king of triceps strengtheners, and will give you elbows forged from steel. Get into a regular pushup position, and smoothly bend the elbows until your forearms are flat on the floor—like a tiger. From here, use arm strength to solidly press yourself back to the start. Many old school strongmen used to perform tiger bends from a handstand position!

CONVICT CONDITIONING — ULTIMATE BODYWEIGHT TRAINING LOG

DAY: _____
DATE: _____

NO.	EXERCISE	SET 1	SET 2	SET 3	SET 4	SET 5

EXTRAS:

COMMENTS:

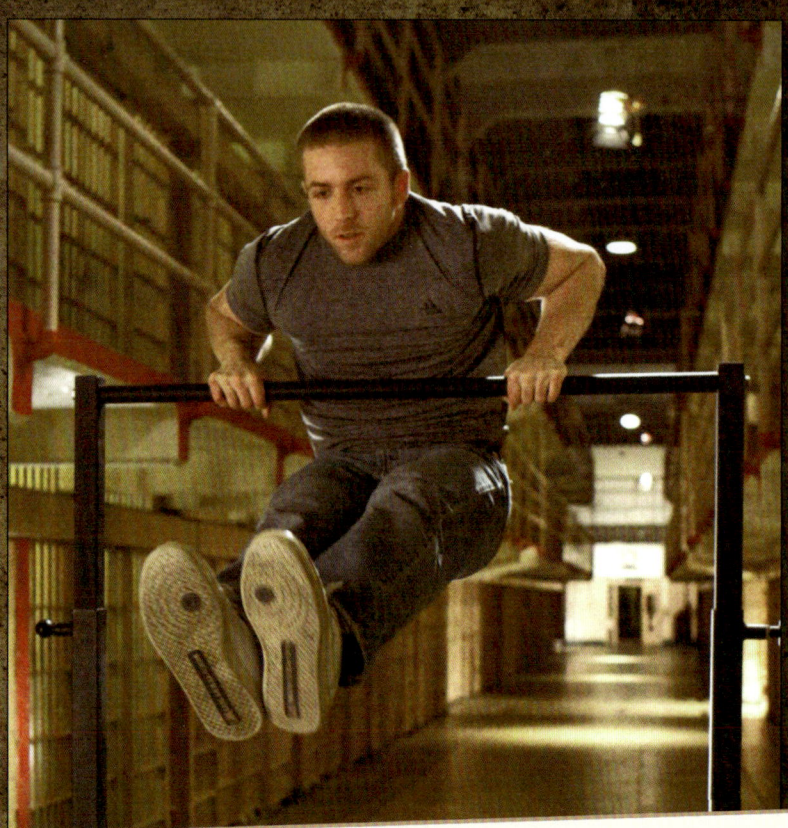

ON PROGRESS:

Despite what some folks will tell ya, strength training really isn't like running in a straight line, where you make dramatic progress continually. *It's more like trying to walk while juggling*. Athletes are juggling all the time—juggling injuries, stress, overwork, low motivation, viruses, biorhythms, lack of rest and similar junk that makes up what we call "life". Two steps forward, one step back is cool.

PAUL "COACH" WADE'S CONVICT CONDITIONING — ULTIMATE BODYWEIGHT TRAINING LOG

DAY: _____

DATE: _____

NO.	EXERCISE	SET 1	SET 2	SET 3	SET 4	SET 5

EXTRAS:

COMMENTS:

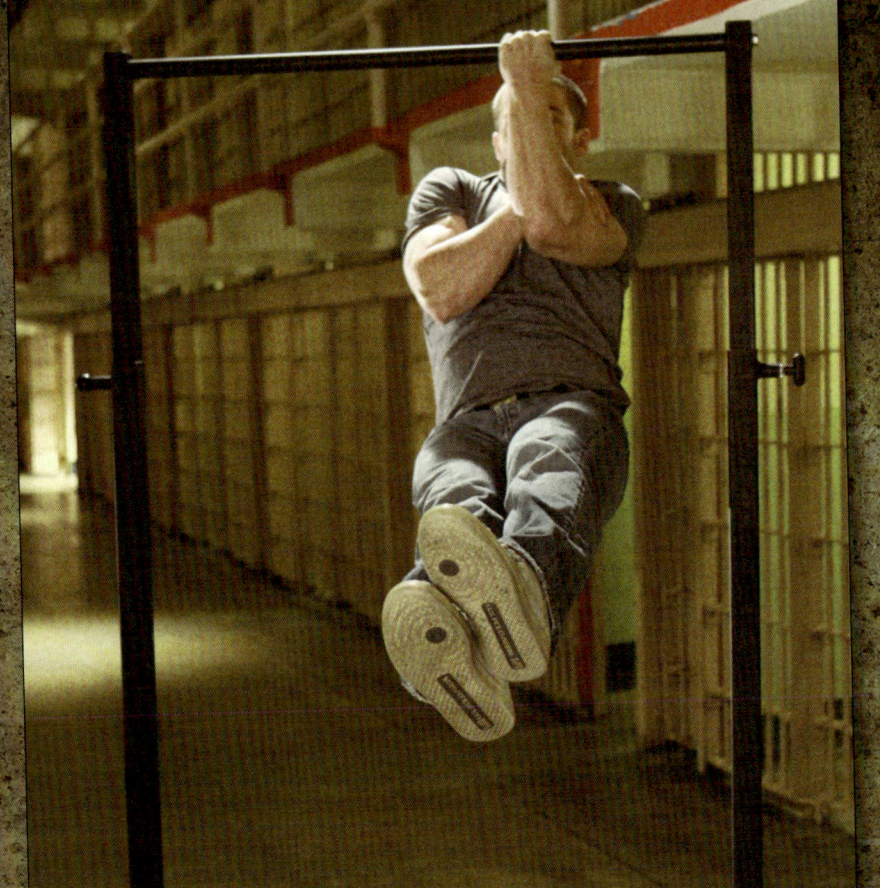

On hard training:

I see a lot of people training who are afraid to really push their bodies *hard*—as if hard work will damage them. This is not right; once you are conditioned, you should push yourself hard when you train. Your muscles aren't like disposable razors which only have so many uses in them: they are more like cellphone batteries—if you want to extend their life, drain them fully before they charge back up.

CONVICT CONDITIONING
Ultimate Bodyweight Training Log

DAY: _____

DATE: _____

167

NO.	EXERCISE	SET 1	SET 2	SET 3	SET 4	SET 5

EXTRAS:

COMMENTS:

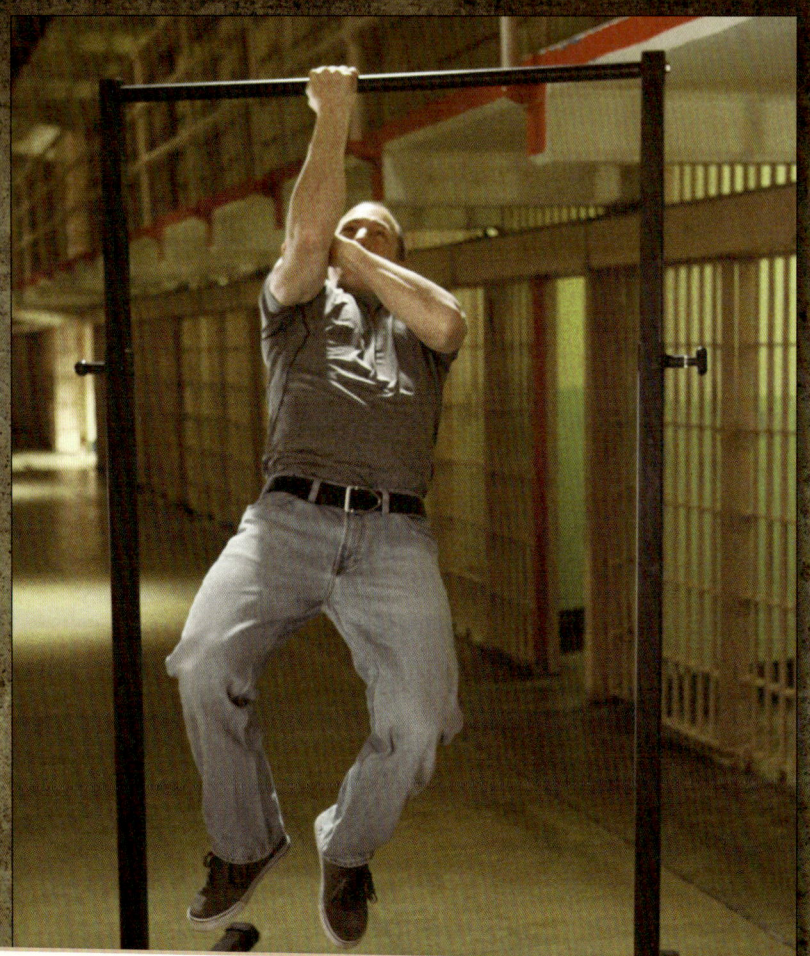

ON REST-PAUSE:

If you want to really work your muscles hard without pushing an exercise to failure, try the *rest-pause method*. Work an exercise until you have maybe two, three reps left. Then pause and take a ten second break, before performing another single rep. Pause again, and perform a second single. You can often get another six or seven near-perfect reps this way—no failure required.

CONVICT CONDITIONING — ULTIMATE BODYWEIGHT TRAINING LOG

DAY: _____
DATE: _____

NO.	EXERCISE	SET 1	SET 2	SET 3	SET 4	SET 5

EXTRAS:

COMMENTS:

ON PARTIALS:

To give their muscles a little extra jolt of work, many bodyweight athletes I have trained with perform "partial reps" at the end of a set. These were called "burns" back in the fifties and sixties. Just complete your set with full range reps as you normally would, but immediately follow up with another three or four reps only going half (or 1/3rd) of the way back down. This hits the muscle tissues very deeply.

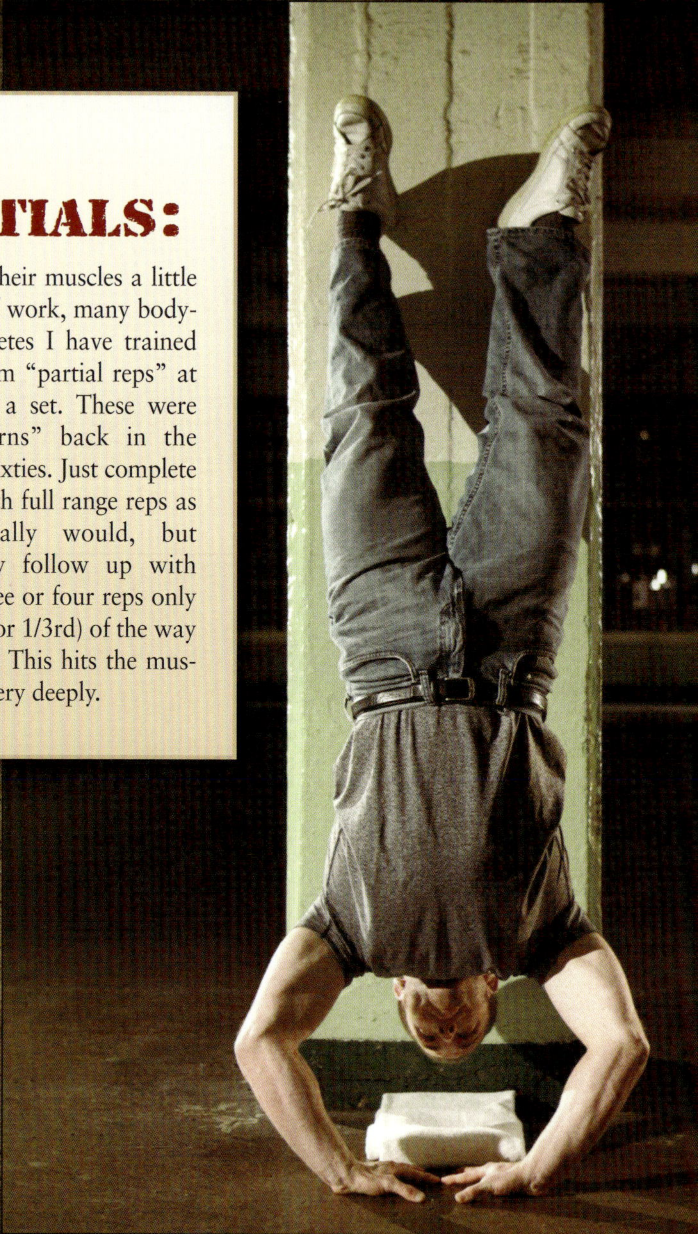

CONVICT CONDITIONING — Ultimate Bodyweight TRAINING LOG

DAY: _____

DATE: _____

NO.	EXERCISE	SET 1	SET 2	SET 3	SET 4	SET 5

EXTRAS:

COMMENTS:

On Calf Training:

The calf muscles are incredibly powerful muscles—second only to the jaw muscles for proportional strength. They can lift huge weights, but calf machines put this weight through the spine or knees, causing compression and joint pain. If you want to test your calves' true power, go with nature. Don't use *weight*: use *velocity*. Explosive jumping and sprinting works the calf muscles better than any machine in the world.

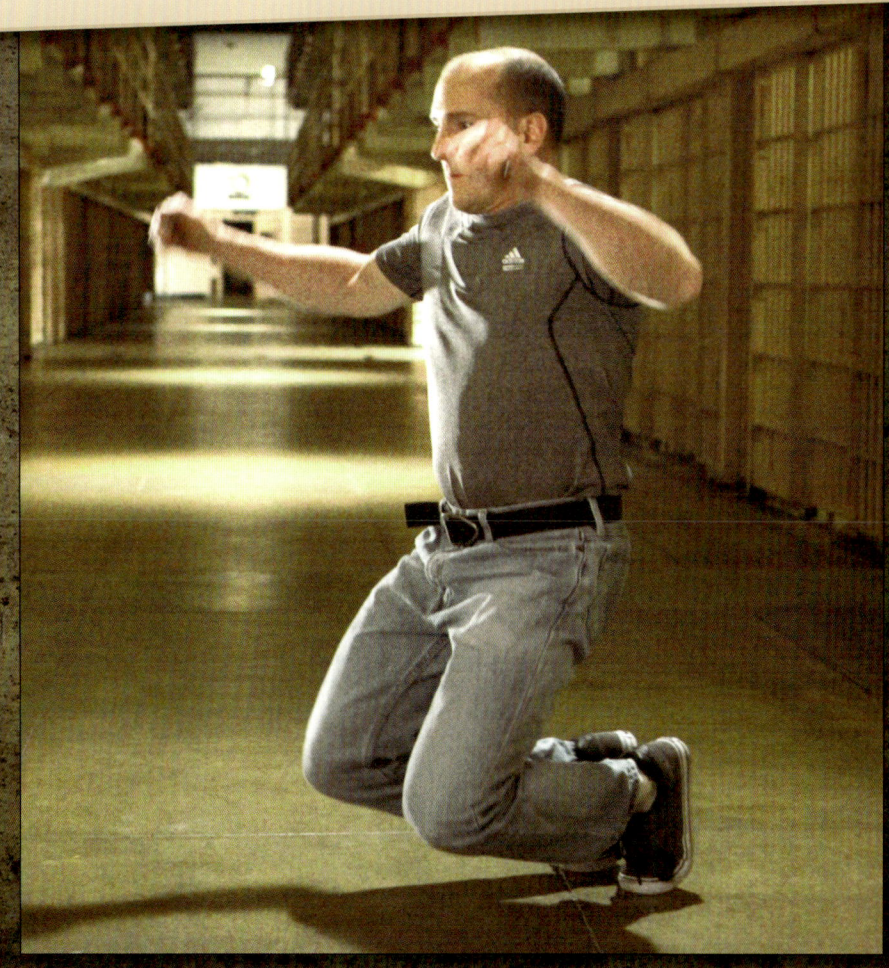

PAUL "COACH" WADE'S CONVICT CONDITIONING
ULTIMATE BODYWEIGHT TRAINING LOG

DAY: _____
DATE: _____

NO.	EXERCISE	SET 1	SET 2	SET 3	SET 4	SET 5

EXTRAS:

COMMENTS:

ON HANDSTANDS:

At some point every calisthenics athlete should explore free handstands—also known as *hand balancing*. Once you are comfortable with wall handstands, begin to gently push your feet an inch or two from the wall. Once you can hold yourself "free" for 30 seconds, try kicking into a handstand in the center of the room. Be ready to safely roll out if you have to!

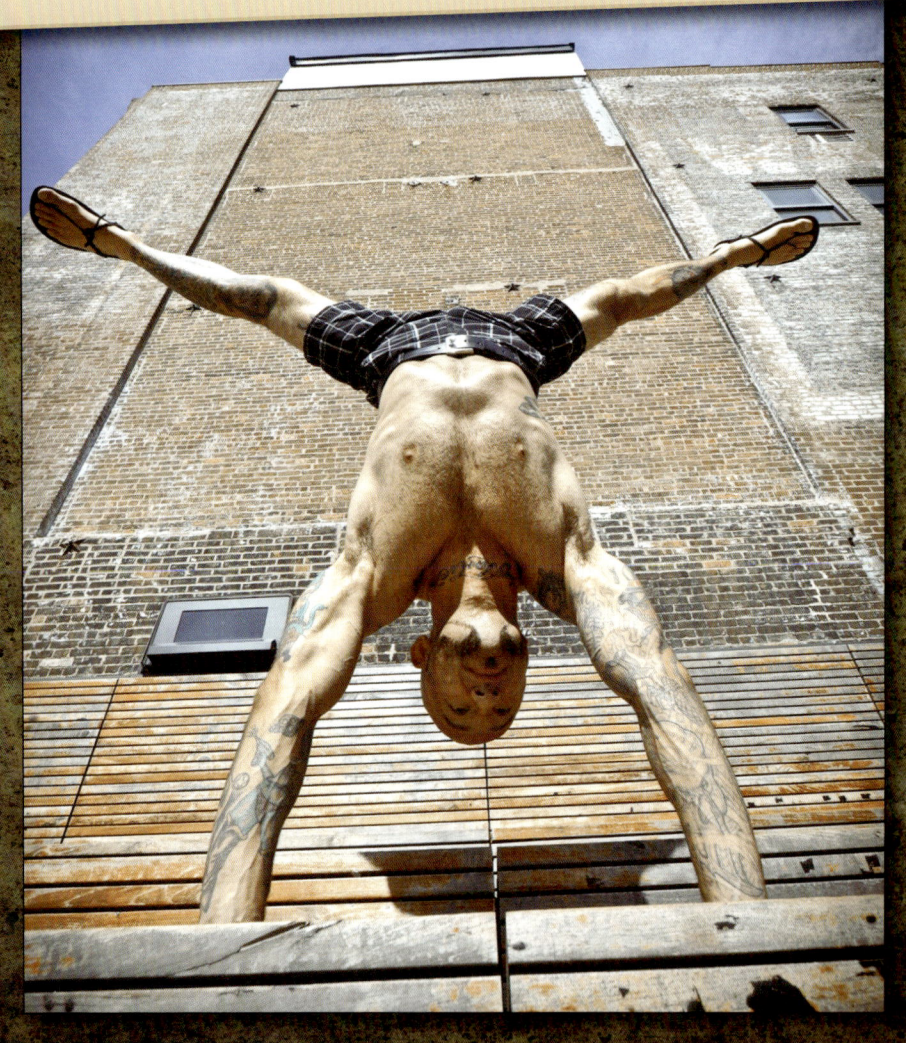

PAUL "COACH" WADE'S CONVICT CONDITIONING
ULTIMATE BODYWEIGHT TRAINING LOG

DAY: _____
DATE: _____

NO.	EXERCISE	SET 1	SET 2	SET 3	SET 4	SET 5

EXTRAS:

COMMENTS:

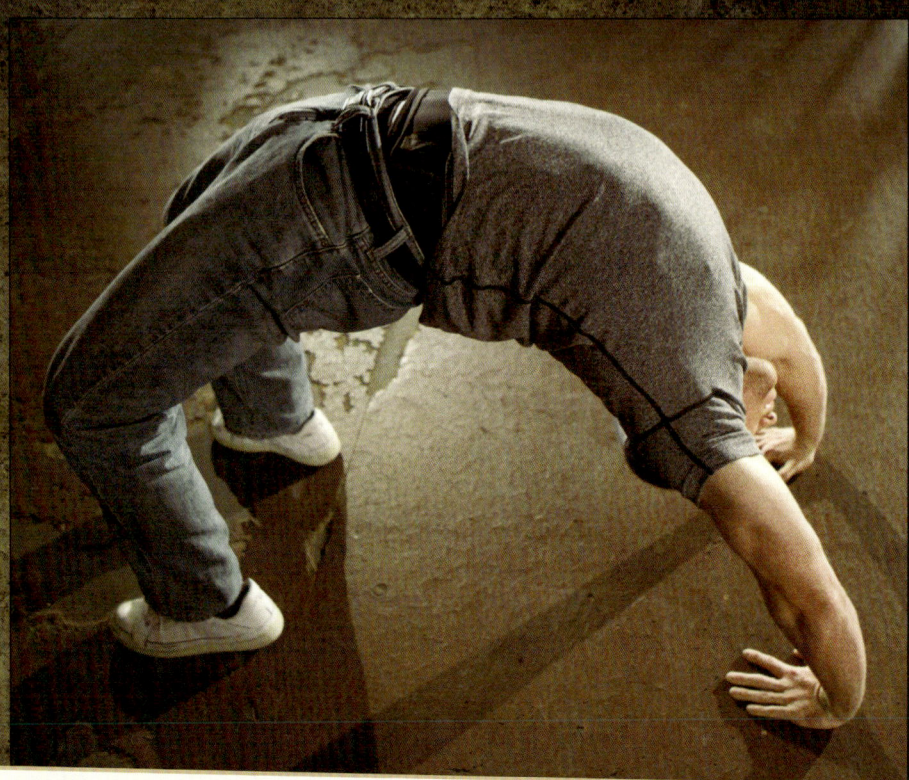

On Natural Cycling:

Unlike weight-training, progressive bodyweight training naturally encourages you to cycle your training efforts. When you begin working with an exercise, you struggle to perform lower reps, and gain more strength and tendon power. As you move toward higher reps over time, you are building endurance and cardiovascular energy. You eventually graduate onto a new, more difficult exercise and the lower rep work begins once more.

CONVICT CONDITIONING — ULTIMATE BODYWEIGHT TRAINING LOG

DAY: _____
DATE: _____

NO.	EXERCISE	SET 1	SET 2	SET 3	SET 4	SET 5

EXTRAS:

COMMENTS:

On sleep:

I have been asked several times whether there is a natural alternative to anabolic steroids. Having worked with many, many different athletes in prison—where inmates sleep and rest much longer than the average stiff—I can say without a doubt that *sleep* is the closest thing there is to a steroid alternative. I'm not one of these "you can sleep too much" people. Nobody I work with on the outside sleeps enough to fulfill their potential. *You* aren't sleeping enough. Sleep more!

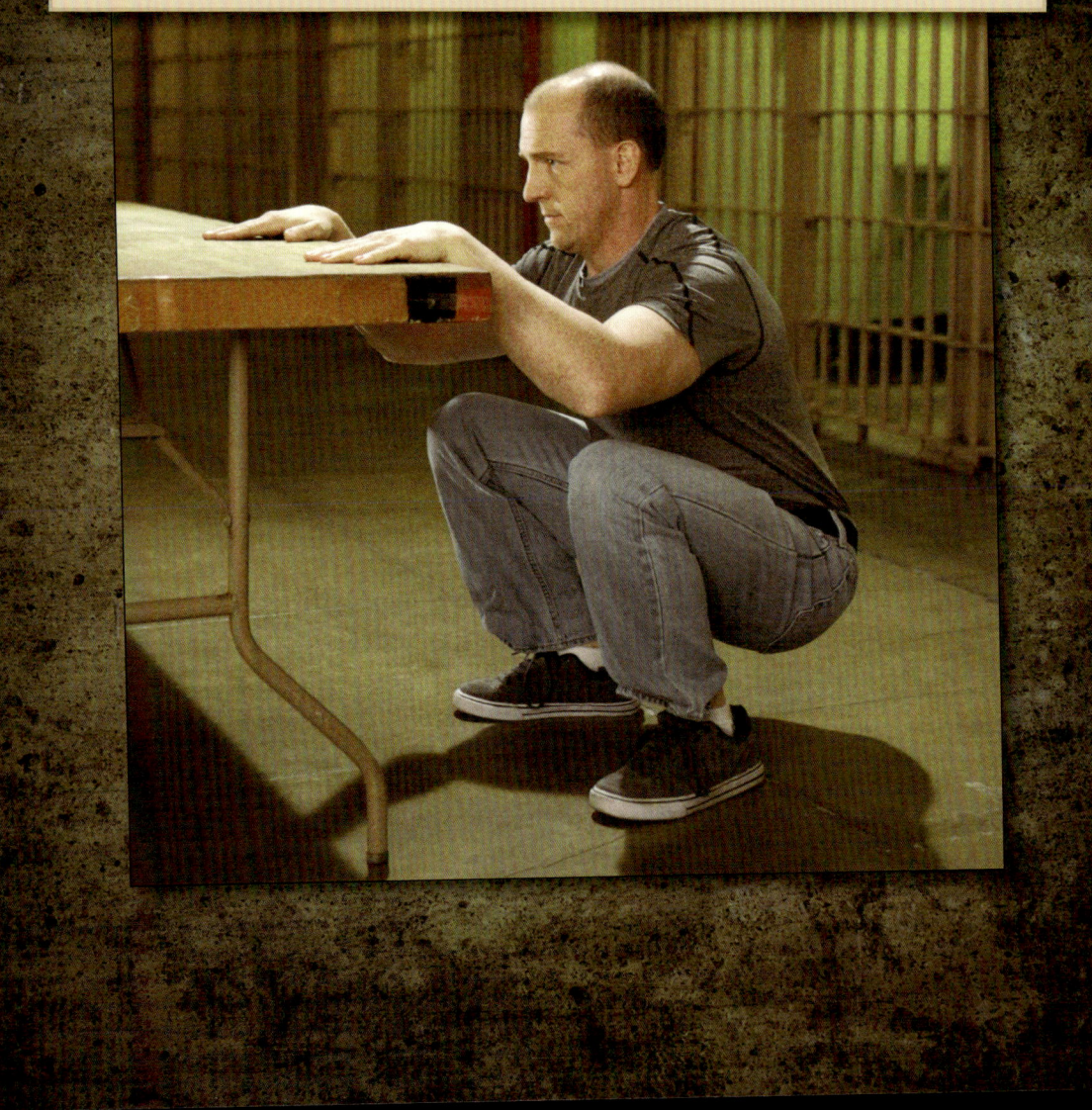

CONVICT CONDITIONING — Ultimate Bodyweight TRAINING LOG

DAY: _____

DATE: _____

NO.	EXERCISE	SET 1	SET 2	SET 3	SET 4	SET 5

EXTRAS:

COMMENTS:

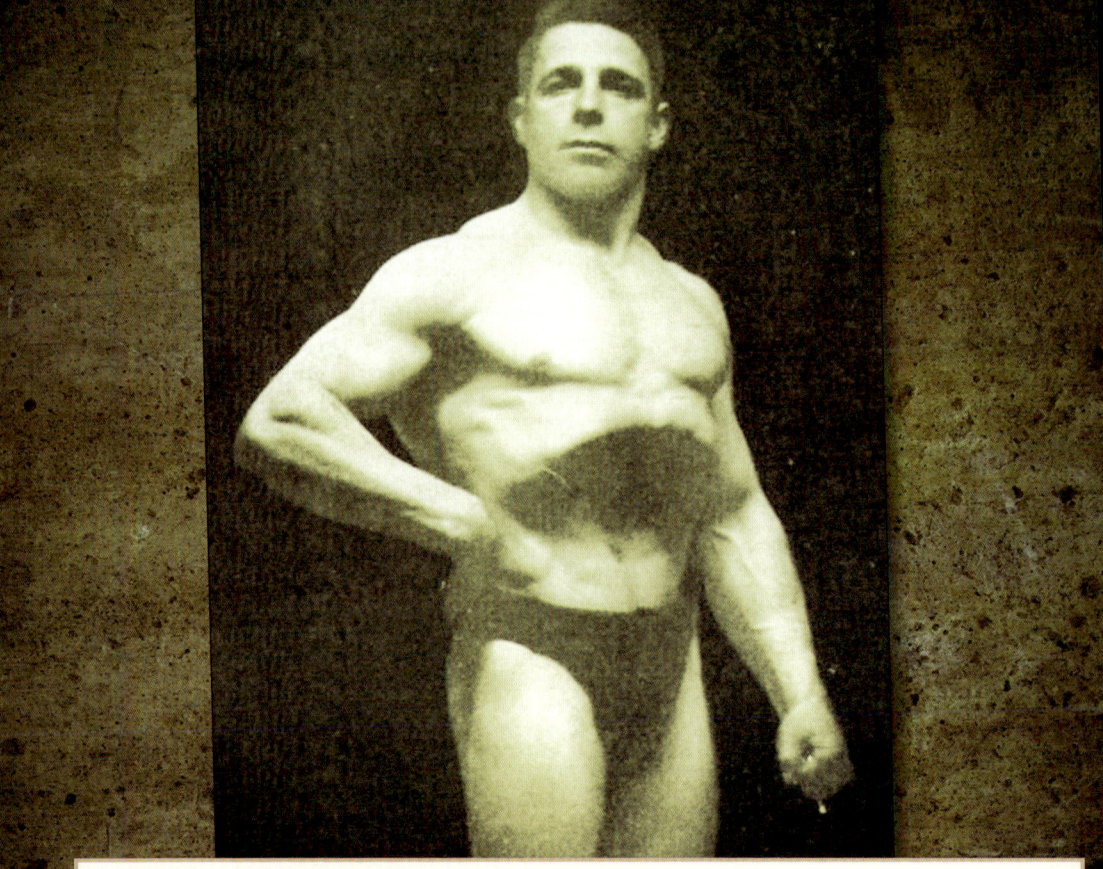

ON CHEST TRAINING:

Former generations of calisthenics masters like Maxick (above) understood that training the chest is about more than having "big pecs". You should also train the important (but less showy) intercostals (muscles of the ribcage) and diaphragm. You can do this by focusing on full, dynamic inhalation and exhalation during training; you can also round off your training session with deep breathing exercises. This will not only strengthen the diaphragm and ribcage, it will also massage the internal organs and detoxify the blood after exertion.

CONVICT CONDITIONING — Ultimate Bodyweight TRAINING LOG

DAY: _____

DATE: _____

NO.	EXERCISE	SET 1	SET 2	SET 3	SET 4	SET 5

EXTRAS:

COMMENTS:

On the training "week":

Remember when you check out workout plans that they are usually built around a seven-day week. This is misleading. The body knows night and day, and rest and activity—it doesn't recognize a "week". If you need to cut a day from the seven-day workout plan, do it. If you need to add a day, or two, do it. If you can't do pullups on Monday, but can hit them on Tuesday, do it. There is nothing sacred about the idea of a "week".

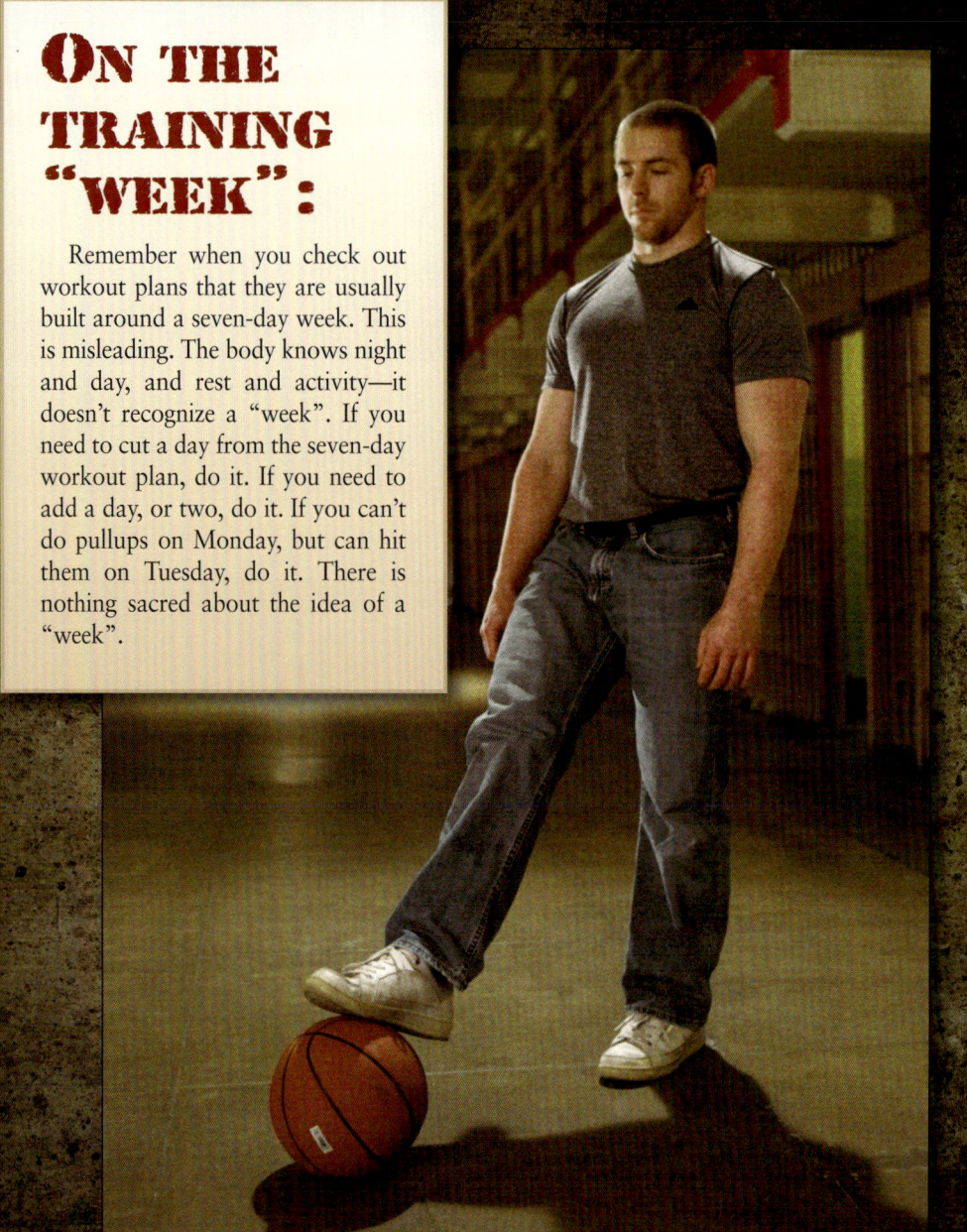

PAUL "COACH" WADE'S CONVICT CONDITIONING — Ultimate Bodyweight Training Log

DAY: _____
DATE: _____

NO.	EXERCISE	SET 1	SET 2	SET 3	SET 4	SET 5

EXTRAS:

COMMENTS:

On Shin Training:

Lots of athletes work their calf muscles (the *gastrocnemius* and *soleus*) but very few work the muscles at the front of the lower leg: the shins (*anterior tibialis*). The best basic exercise for tibialis training is the one-leg squat—hands down! Try it, while holding onto something. After just a few reps, the shin muscles begin to burn under the powerful pressure of fixing the feet in the necessary position.

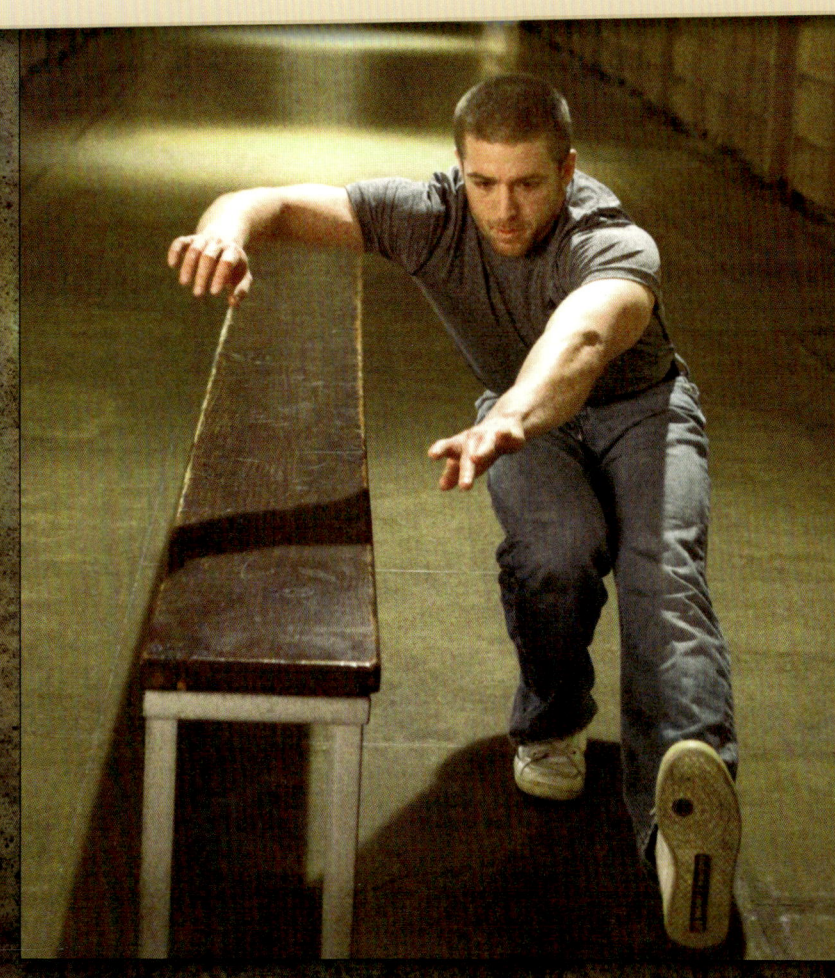

CONVICT CONDITIONING — Ultimate Bodyweight Training Log

DAY: _____

DATE: _____

NO.	EXERCISE	SET 1	SET 2	SET 3	SET 4	SET 5

EXTRAS:

COMMENTS:

ON CROSS-TRAINING:

Never become limited by one form of training—no matter how much you love it. Your body is capable of *millions* of different movements, and you can master *hundreds* of different skills in your lifetime, well into what is called "old age". Build your strength through calisthenics, but learn to *use* that strength somehow, too: box, swim, climb, do yoga, learn martial arts. Use your body to do different things. As obsessed with kung fu as he was, even Bruce Lee learned to dance the cha-cha-cha. (He became a champion at it.)

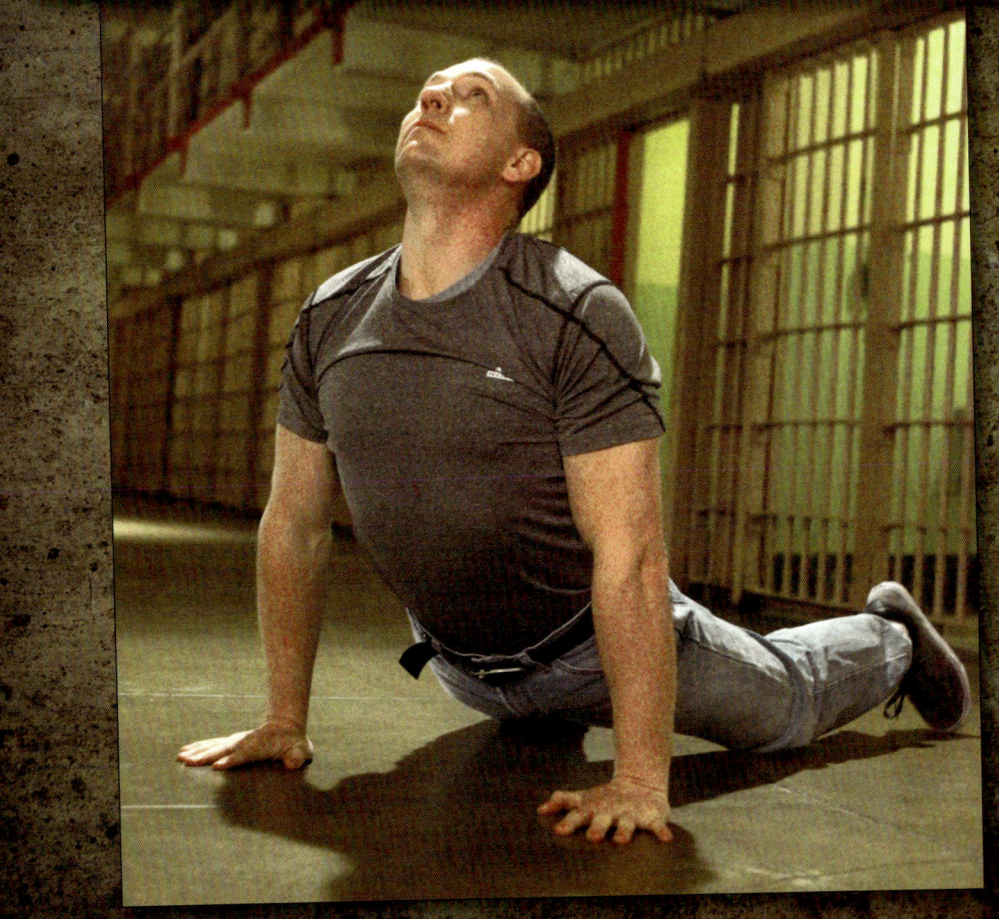

CONVICT CONDITIONING ULTIMATE BODYWEIGHT TRAINING LOG

DAY: _____
DATE: _____

NO.	EXERCISE	SET 1	SET 2	SET 3	SET 4	SET 5

EXTRAS:

COMMENTS:

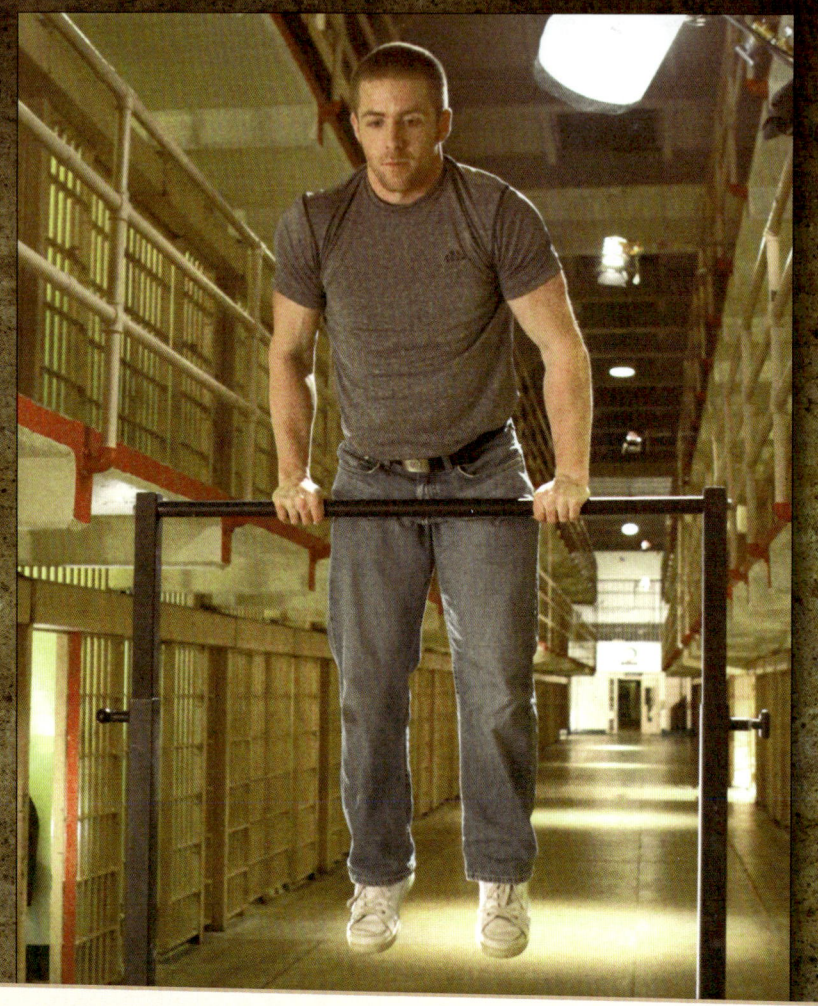

ON PECS:

Looking for a jolt of extra muscle in your pecs? A secret weapon for huge pecs is the *bar dip*. Get above an overhead bar, dip until your sternum touches the bar, and push back up. Most body-weight athletes are familiar with dips on the parallel bars, but parallel dips make you keep your hands to your *sides*, and this allows the lats help in the press. During bar dips, your hands are forced in *front* of you, and the pecs have to do more of the work, resulting in extra growth.

PAUL "COACH" WADE'S CONVICT CONDITIONING — Ultimate Bodyweight Training Log

DAY: _____
DATE: _____

NO.	EXERCISE	SET 1	SET 2	SET 3	SET 4	SET 5

EXTRAS:

COMMENTS:

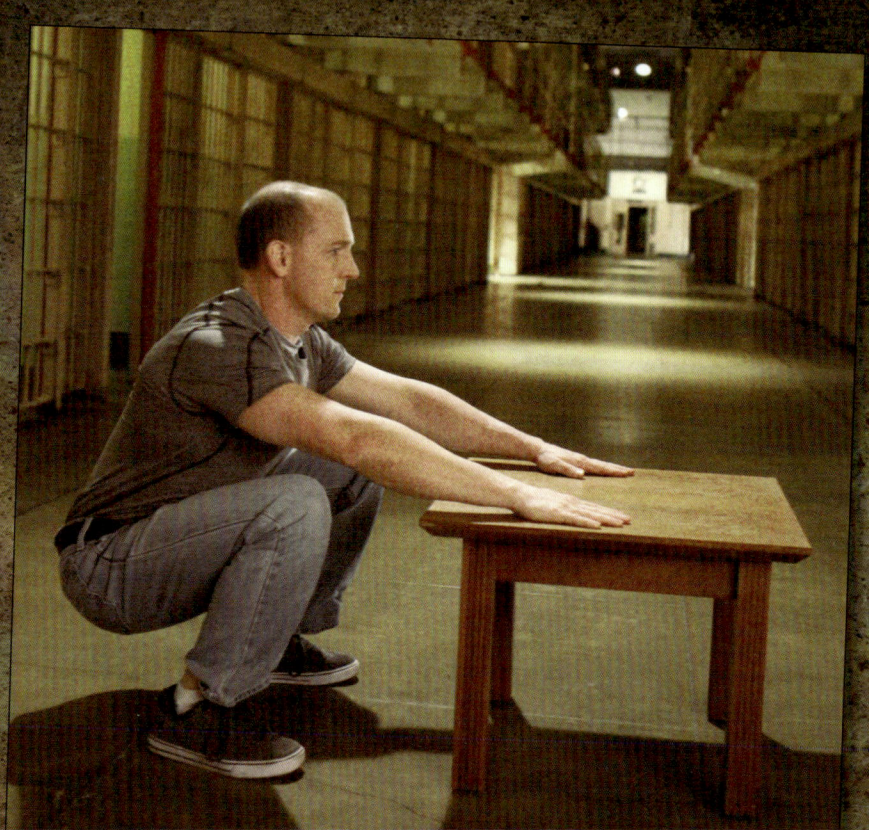

ON BOARD SQUATTING:

Squatting with the heels up can damage the knees. I've seen lots of folks place boards under their heels when they squat; they claim that "due to their structure" they cannot squat flat-footed. This is bull! Inability to perform a good squat has nothing to do with structure, and everything to do with poor ankle mobility. Learn to squat flat-footed by investing time in deep squatting exercises like *jackknife squats* and *supported squats,* and you will never need to use a board.

PAUL "COACH" WADE'S CONVICT CONDITIONING — Ultimate Bodyweight Training Log

DAY: _____

DATE: _____

NO.	EXERCISE	SET 1	SET 2	SET 3	SET 4	SET 5

EXTRAS:

COMMENTS:

On Deltoids:

The deltoid has three heads, joining together to make up a large "D" shape when viewed from the top (Delta is the Greek letter "D"). Giving any of the heads extra stimulation is easy—just use a wider hand placement during your exercises. *Wide pullups* hit the rear delts hard; *wide pushups* hit the front delts; and a wider hand placement on *handstands* will hit the side delts like a runaway train.

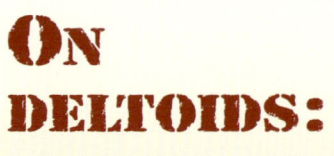

PAUL "COACH" WADE'S CONVICT CONDITIONING ULTIMATE BODYWEIGHT TRAINING LOG

DAY: _____
DATE: _____

NO.	EXERCISE	SET 1	SET 2	SET 3	SET 4	SET 5

EXTRAS:

COMMENTS:

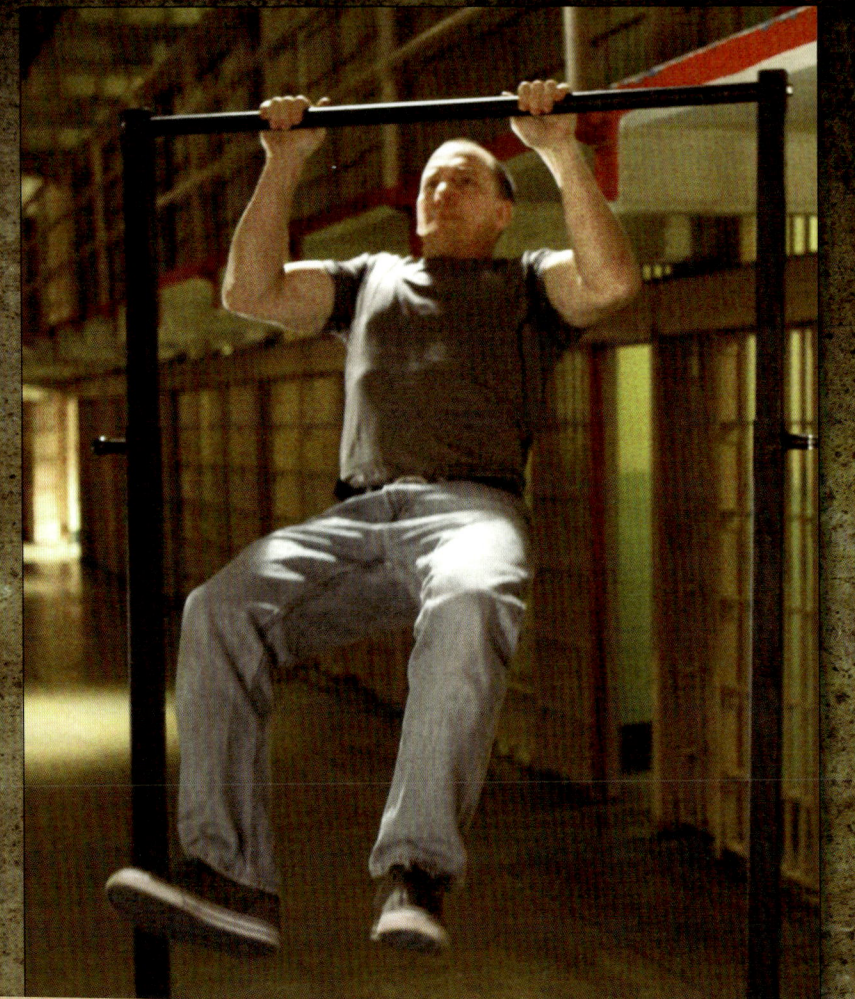

ON HYLAND'S RECORD:

After years of injury and inactivity, Stephen Hyland began working out at age 43. Calisthenics revolutionized the man. In 2010, Hyland broke his own record by performing 1009 pullups in a single hour. Hey…you can build up to a *tenth* of that, right?

CONVICT CONDITIONING — Ultimate Bodyweight TRAINING LOG

DAY: _____

DATE: _____

NO.	EXERCISE	SET 1	SET 2	SET 3	SET 4	SET 5

EXTRAS:

COMMENTS:

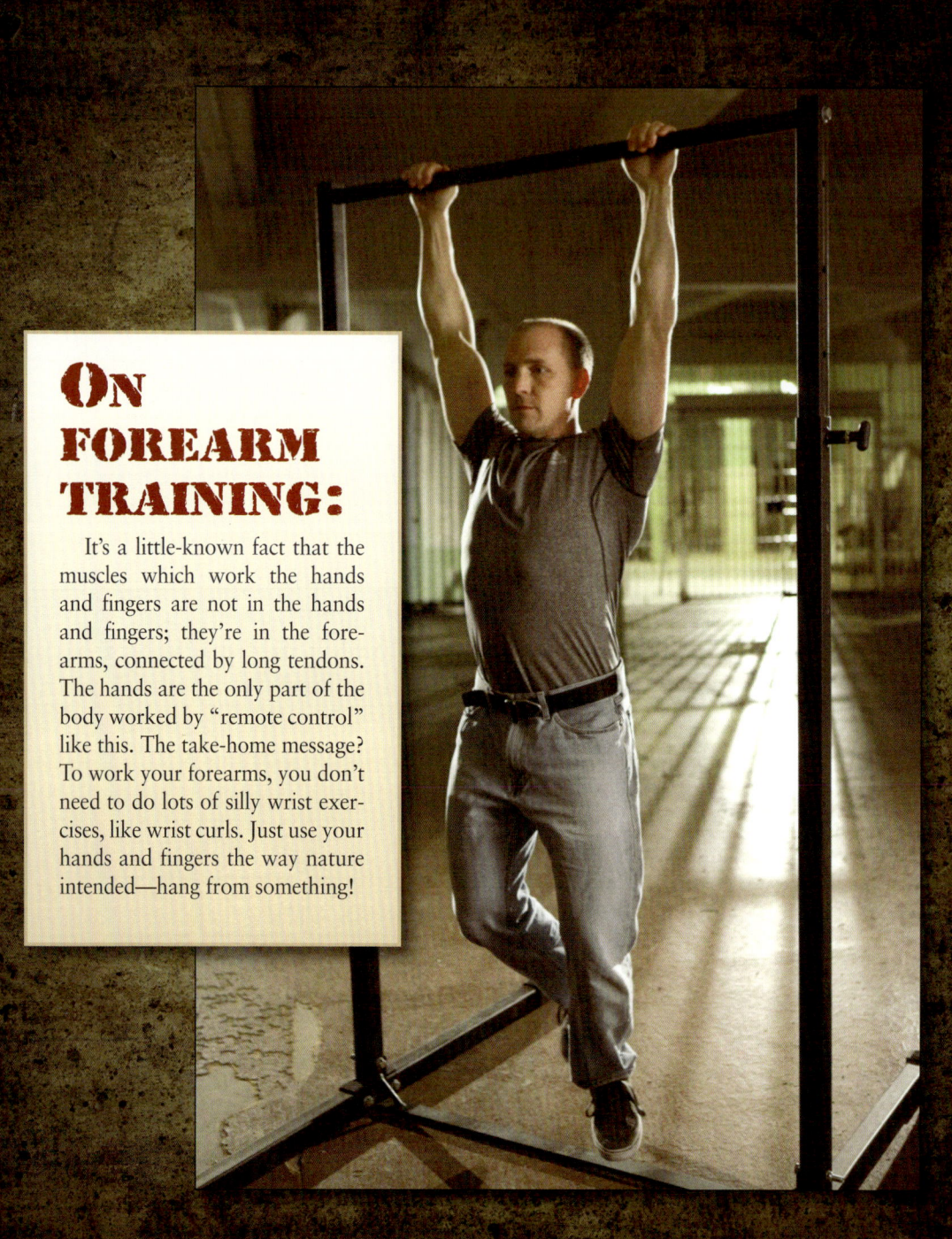

ON FOREARM TRAINING:

It's a little-known fact that the muscles which work the hands and fingers are not in the hands and fingers; they're in the forearms, connected by long tendons. The hands are the only part of the body worked by "remote control" like this. The take-home message? To work your forearms, you don't need to do lots of silly wrist exercises, like wrist curls. Just use your hands and fingers the way nature intended—hang from something!

PAUL "COACH" WADE'S CONVICT CONDITIONING
Ultimate Bodyweight Training Log

DAY: _____
DATE: _____

NO.	EXERCISE	SET 1	SET 2	SET 3	SET 4	SET 5

EXTRAS:

COMMENTS:

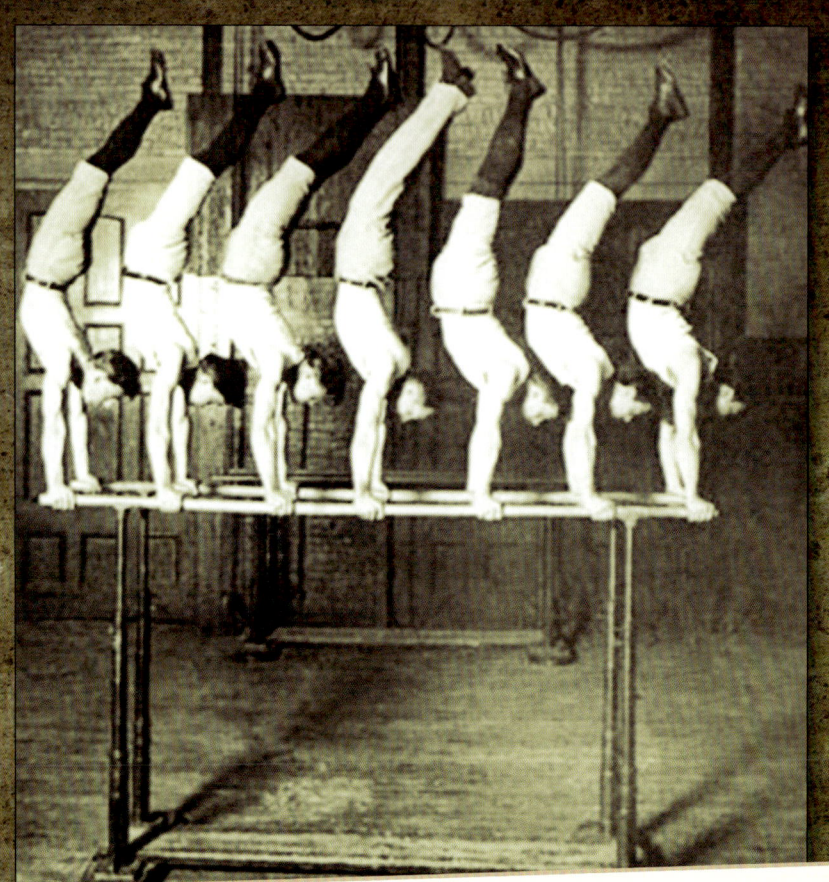

ON VERTICAL WORK:

Ancient systems of gymnastics all included some kind of training on a *vertical column* or pole, to develop the lateral muscles of the body so useful for combat. When Friedrich Ludwig Jahn formalized European gymnastics in the 19th century, he sadly left out vertical apparatus, in favor of exclusively horizontal equipment like the parallel bars (above). In the East, vertical column training still survives in the Indian *mallakhamb* and *Chinese pole* disciplines.

PAUL "COACH" WADE'S CONVICT CONDITIONING ULTIMATE BODYWEIGHT TRAINING LOG

DAY: _____

DATE: _____

NO.	EXERCISE	SET 1	SET 2	SET 3	SET 4	SET 5

EXTRAS:

COMMENTS:

ON NECK WORK:

To train the neck properly, you don't need machines and harnesses. Wrestlers have the thickest, strongest necks of any athletes, and this comes from years of neck bridges performed using bodyweight alone. If you want a stronger neck *without* adding any muscle, slowly add time to your headstands. (Five minutes would be a great goal.) Simple headstands, yoga-style, safely strengthen the deep tissue, tendons and vertebrae of the neck over time.

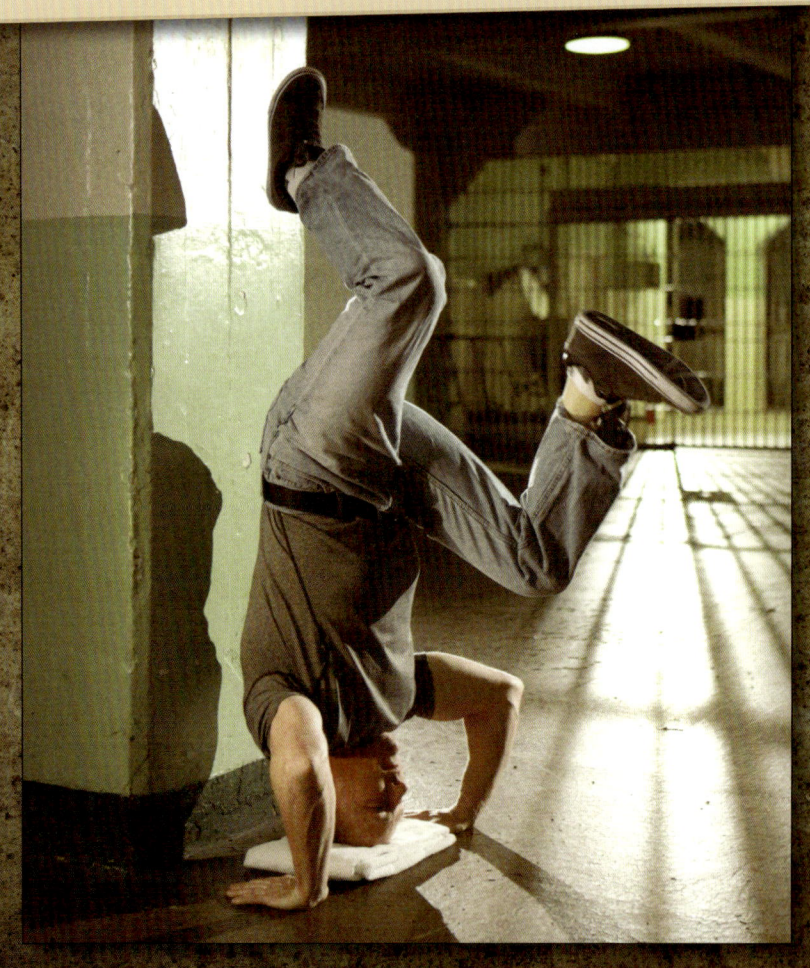

PAUL "COACH" WADE'S CONVICT CONDITIONING
Ultimate Bodyweight Training Log

201

DAY: _____
DATE: _____

NO.	EXERCISE	SET 1	SET 2	SET 3	SET 4	SET 5

EXTRAS:

COMMENTS:

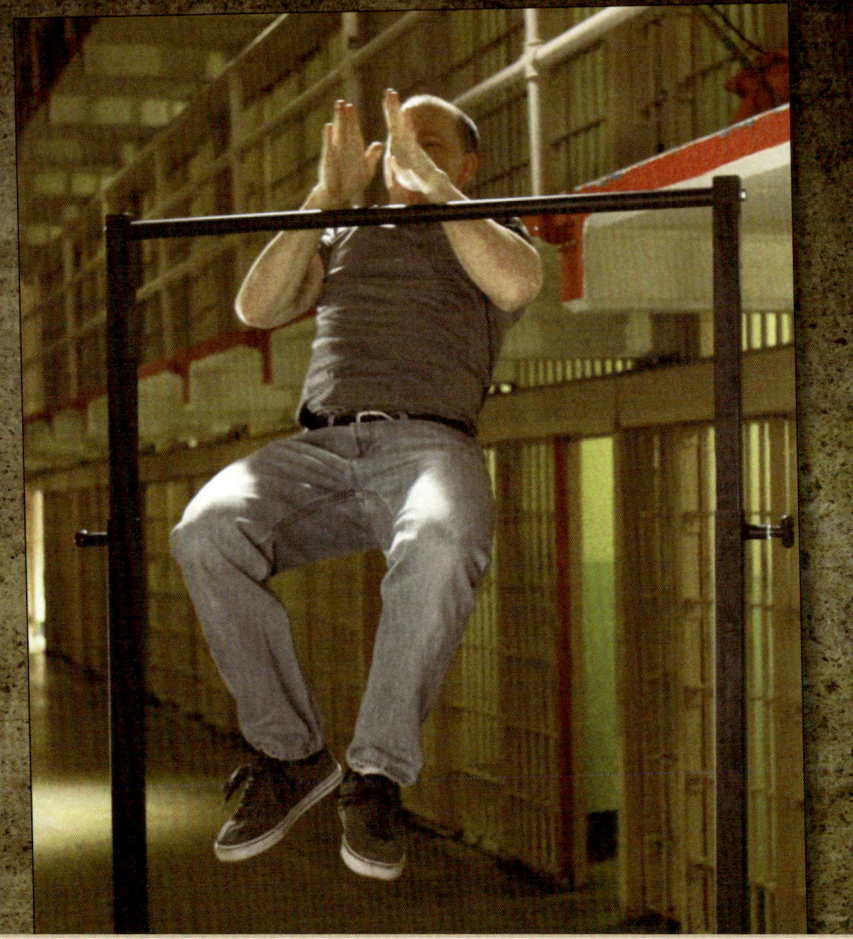

On speed:

Beginners to calisthenics—athletes who cannot perform up to step 5 on pullups, pushups, leg raises and squats—should perform all their exercises slowly and deliberately, to learn the correct body mechanics and strengthen the joints. After this time, some body English can be introduced to your movements. Intermediate and advanced athletes should definitely experiment with faster and even explosive movements from time to time.

PAUL "COACH" WADE'S CONVICT CONDITIONING ULTIMATE BODYWEIGHT TRAINING LOG

DAY: _____

DATE: _____

NO.	EXERCISE	SET 1	SET 2	SET 3	SET 4	SET 5

EXTRAS:

COMMENTS:

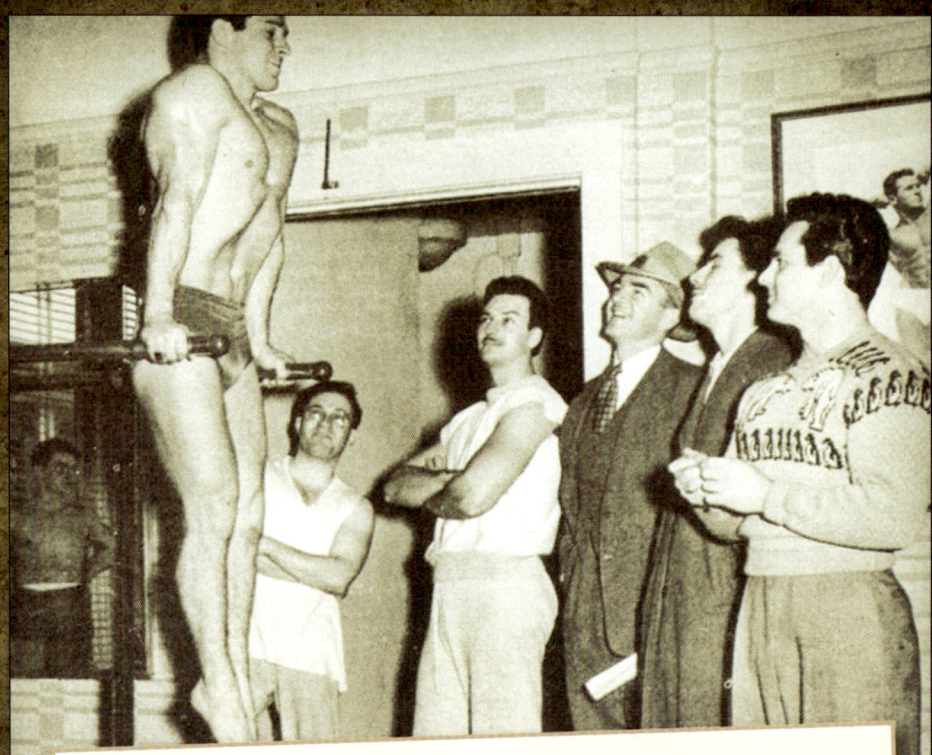

On Jack LaLanne:

Everyone in America knows that Jack LaLanne was in great shape, but fewer know that he was a World Record holder. In 1959 Jack performed an amazing 1000 pushups and 1000 pullups in an hour and 22 minutes! Calisthenics lends itself to training longevity. Jack LaLanne didn't even start breaking bodyweight records until he was well into his forties, by which time most serious athletes have been retired for over a decade.

PAUL "COACH" WADE'S CONVICT CONDITIONING Ultimate Bodyweight Training Log

DAY: _____

DATE: _____

NO.	EXERCISE	SET 1	SET 2	SET 3	SET 4	SET 5

EXTRAS:

COMMENTS:

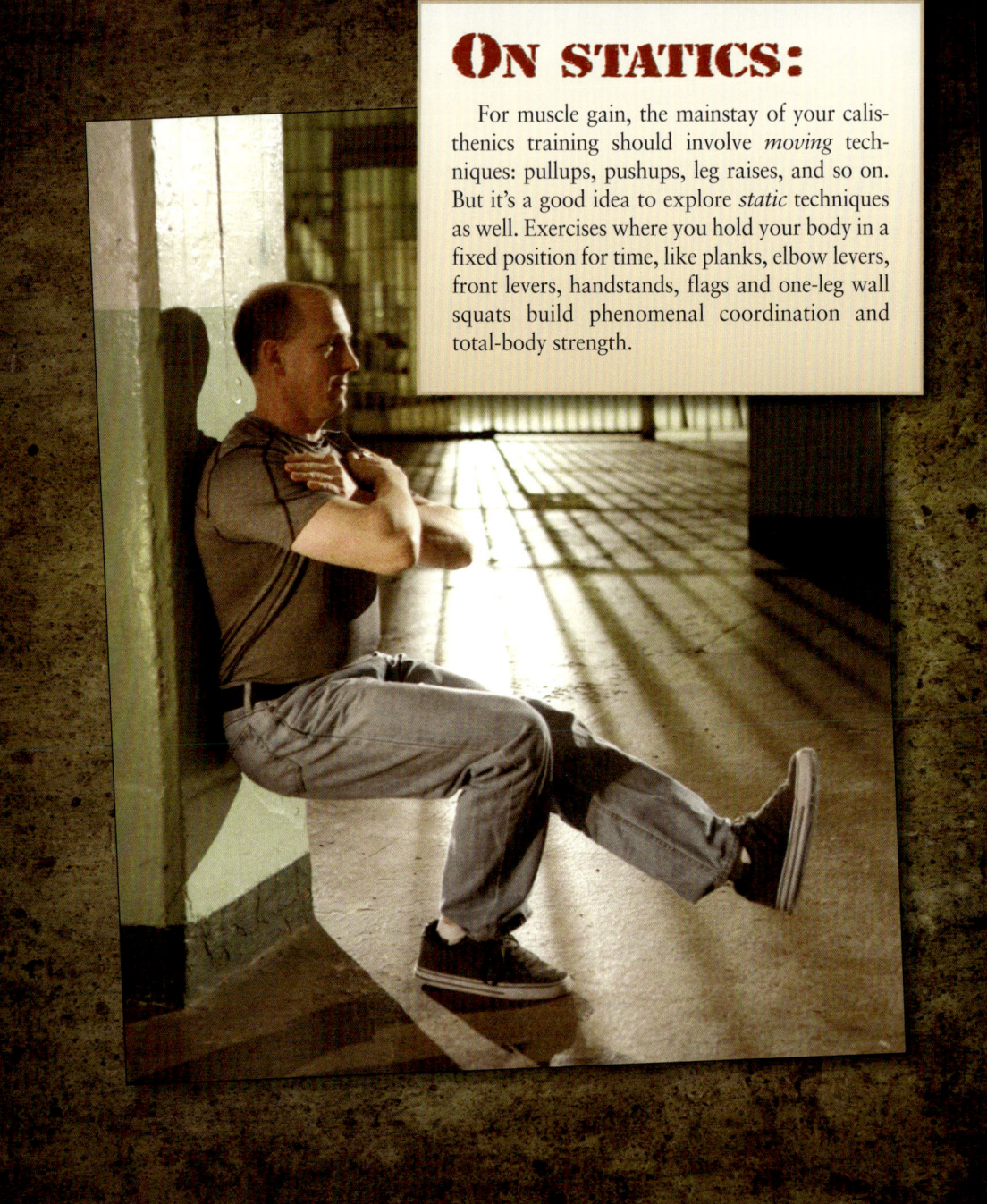

ON STATICS:

For muscle gain, the mainstay of your calisthenics training should involve *moving* techniques: pullups, pushups, leg raises, and so on. But it's a good idea to explore *static* techniques as well. Exercises where you hold your body in a fixed position for time, like planks, elbow levers, front levers, handstands, flags and one-leg wall squats build phenomenal coordination and total-body strength.

PAUL "COACH" WADE'S CONVICT CONDITIONING — Ultimate Bodyweight Training Log

DAY: _____
DATE: _____

NO.	EXERCISE	SET 1	SET 2	SET 3	SET 4	SET 5

EXTRAS:

COMMENTS:

ON CREATIVITY:

The quality most needed for training longevity isn't *discipline* or *willpower*: it's *creativity*. Successful athletes intuitively understand that working out a certain way for too long will leave them burnt-out and lacking motivation. Work diligently at a program for no more than ten weeks max, then change things somehow. No matter how great a routine is, if it's become boring it's doomed. Have fun injecting new ideas, methods and approaches into your training.

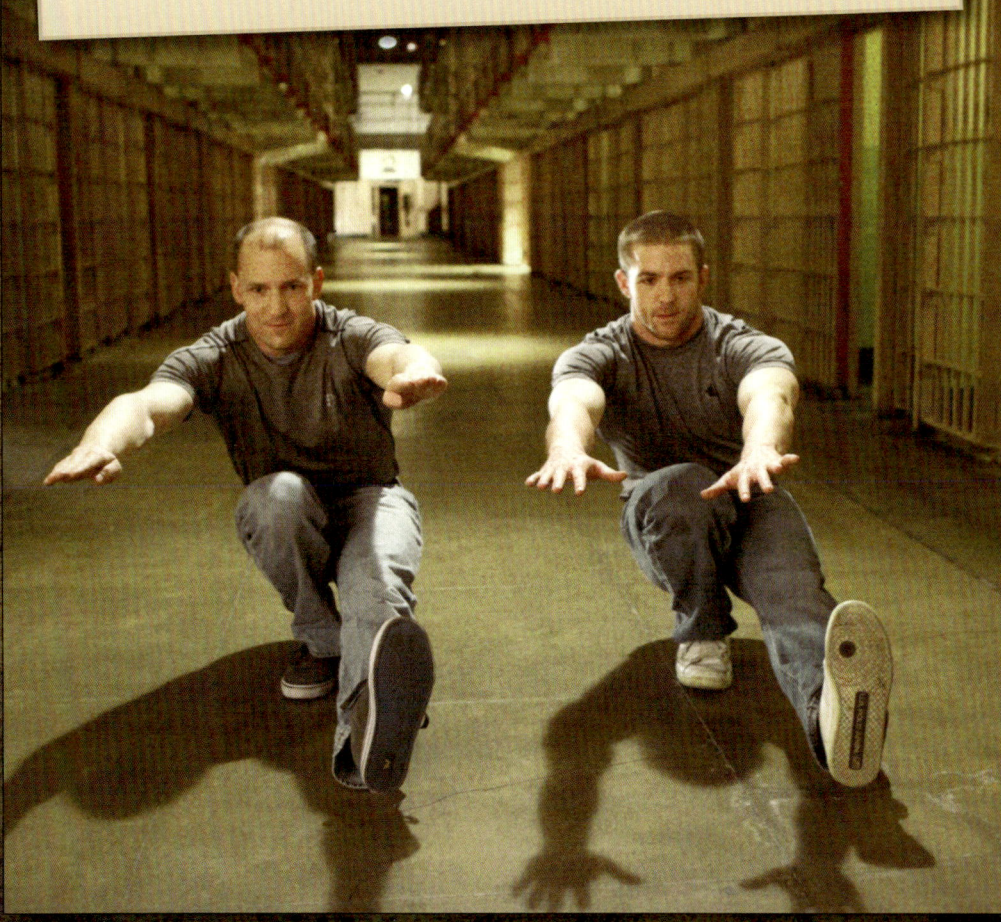

PAUL "COACH" WADE'S CONVICT CONDITIONING — ULTIMATE BODYWEIGHT TRAINING LOG

DAY: _____

DATE: _____

NO.	EXERCISE	SET 1	SET 2	SET 3	SET 4	SET 5

EXTRAS:

COMMENTS:

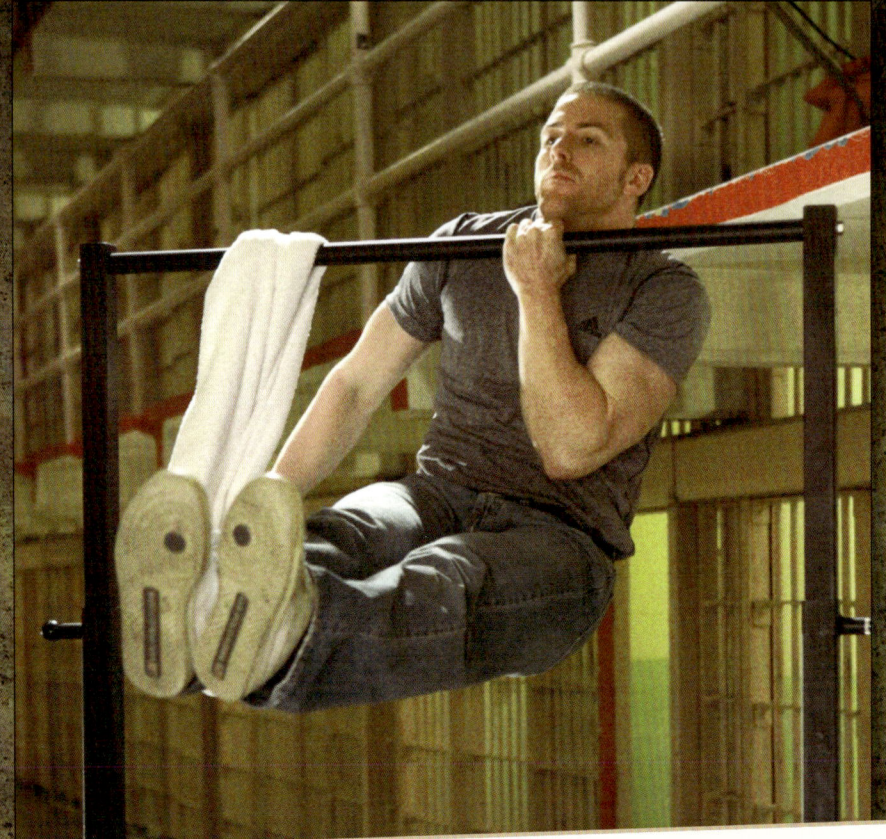

On Consolidation Training:

In most cases when you train on an exercise, it's a good idea to rest a few days before performing that exercise again, to let your muscles recover. But when you encounter techniques that you find just too difficult to get to grips with—because you can't get the technique right, the strength requirements are unusual, or your balance is off—sometimes it's helpful to practice this exercise—just a rep or two—several times throughout the day. This is called *consolidation training*. It will teach your *nervous system* how to perform the technique better, without burning out the *muscles*.

PAUL "COACH" WADE'S CONVICT CONDITIONING
ULTIMATE BODYWEIGHT TRAINING LOG

DAY: _____
DATE: _____

NO.	EXERCISE	SET 1	SET 2	SET 3	SET 4	SET 5

EXTRAS:

COMMENTS:

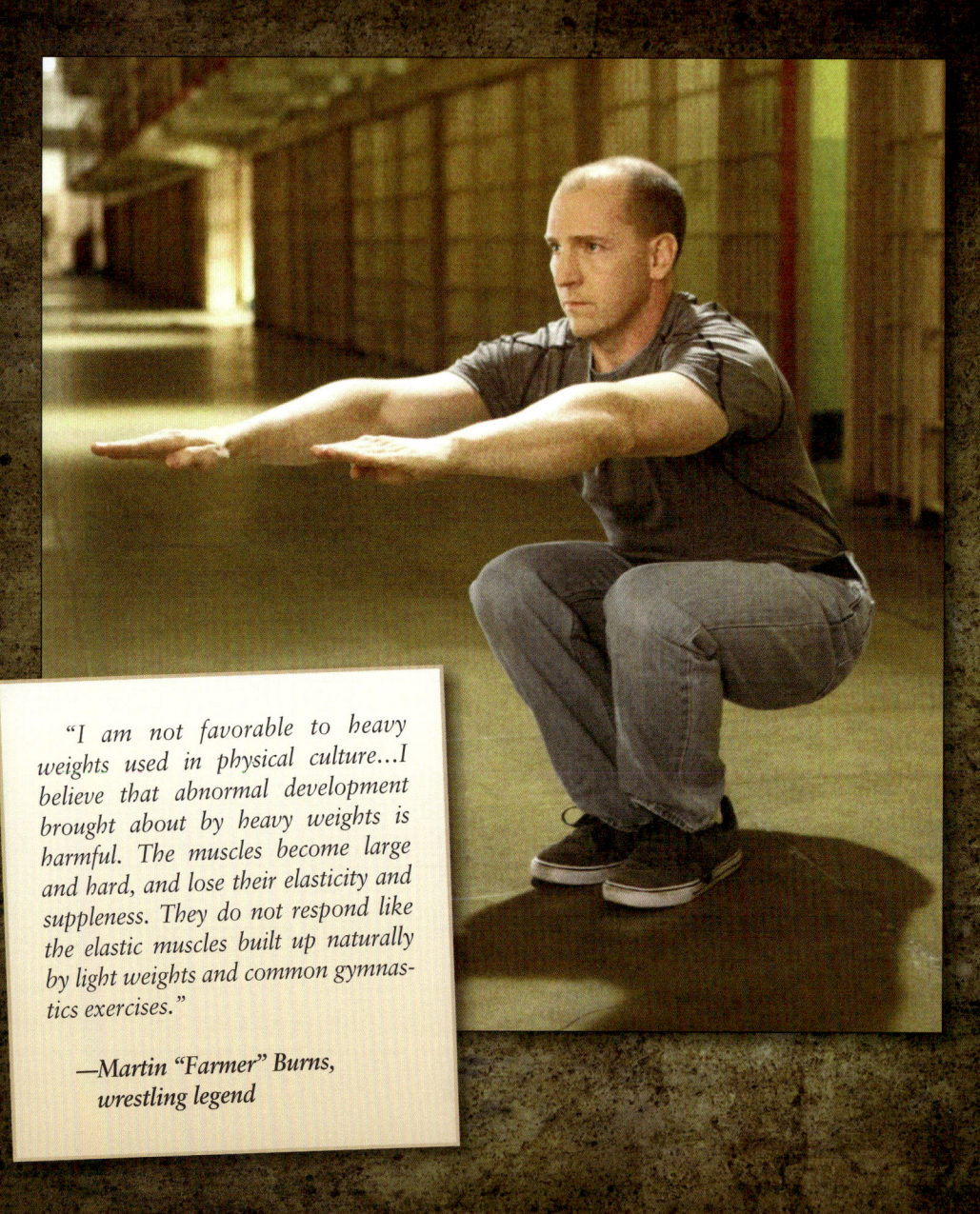

"I am not favorable to heavy weights used in physical culture...I believe that abnormal development brought about by heavy weights is harmful. The muscles become large and hard, and lose their elasticity and suppleness. They do not respond like the elastic muscles built up naturally by light weights and common gymnastics exercises."

—Martin "Farmer" Burns, wrestling legend

PAUL "COACH" WADE'S CONVICT CONDITIONING
Ultimate Bodyweight Training Log

DAY: _____
DATE: _____

NO.	EXERCISE	SET 1	SET 2	SET 3	SET 4	SET 5

EXTRAS:

COMMENTS:

ON EXPLOSIVE TRAINING:

The finest explosive training in the world is *bodyweight-based*. It doesn't require equipment: your body is your gym. Explosive training and agility go hand-in-hand in all athleticism, and training for one develops the other. Can you kip up from the floor? Can you do a cartwheel? Can you do a front flip? Can you perform a sentry pullup? A triple-clap pushup? These moves, and others like them, are the most powerful forms of plyometric training known to man.

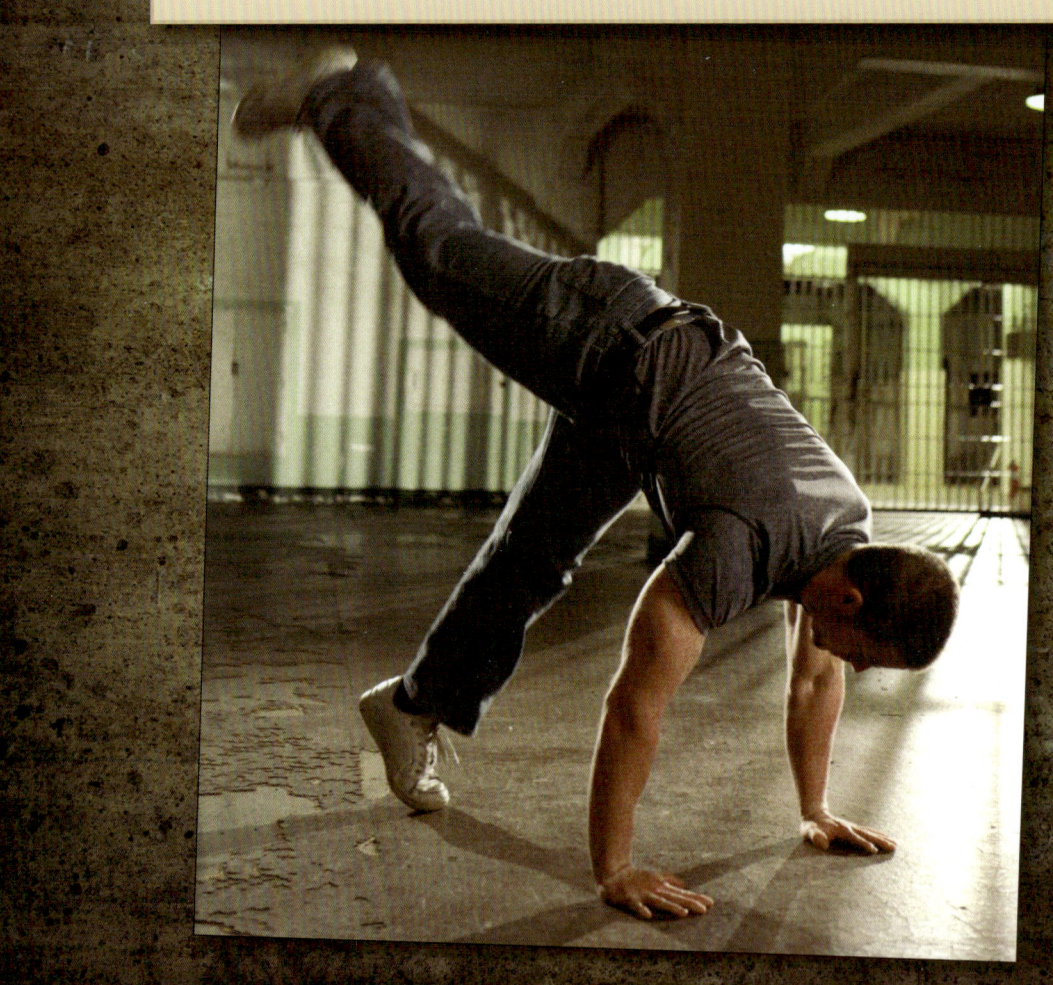

PAUL "COACH" WADE'S CONVICT CONDITIONING ULTIMATE BODYWEIGHT TRAINING LOG

DAY: _____
DATE: _____

NO.	EXERCISE	SET 1	SET 2	SET 3	SET 4	SET 5

EXTRAS:

COMMENTS:

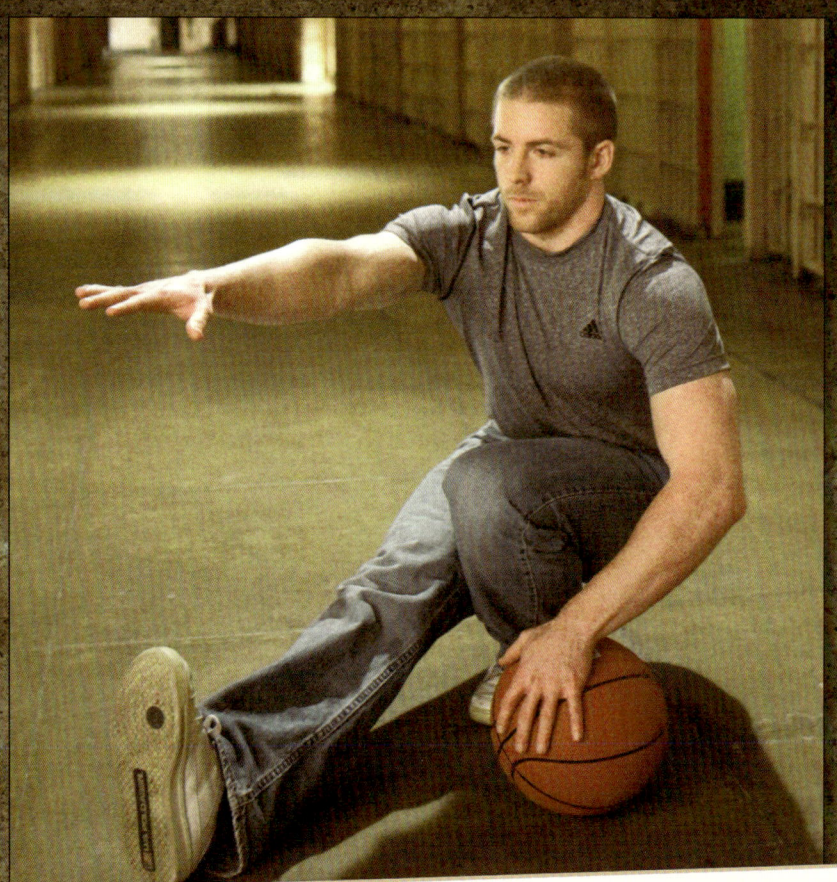

On assistance movements:

Many calisthenics movements are hardest in the bottom position, where the muscles are stretched and at their weakest. In these cases, convicts often use an object—a basketball or a stack of books—to push on to help ease them out of the "hole" without strain.

PAUL "COACH" WADE'S CONVICT CONDITIONING ULTIMATE BODYWEIGHT TRAINING LOG

DAY: _____
DATE: _____

NO.	EXERCISE	SET 1	SET 2	SET 3	SET 4	SET 5

EXTRAS:

COMMENTS:

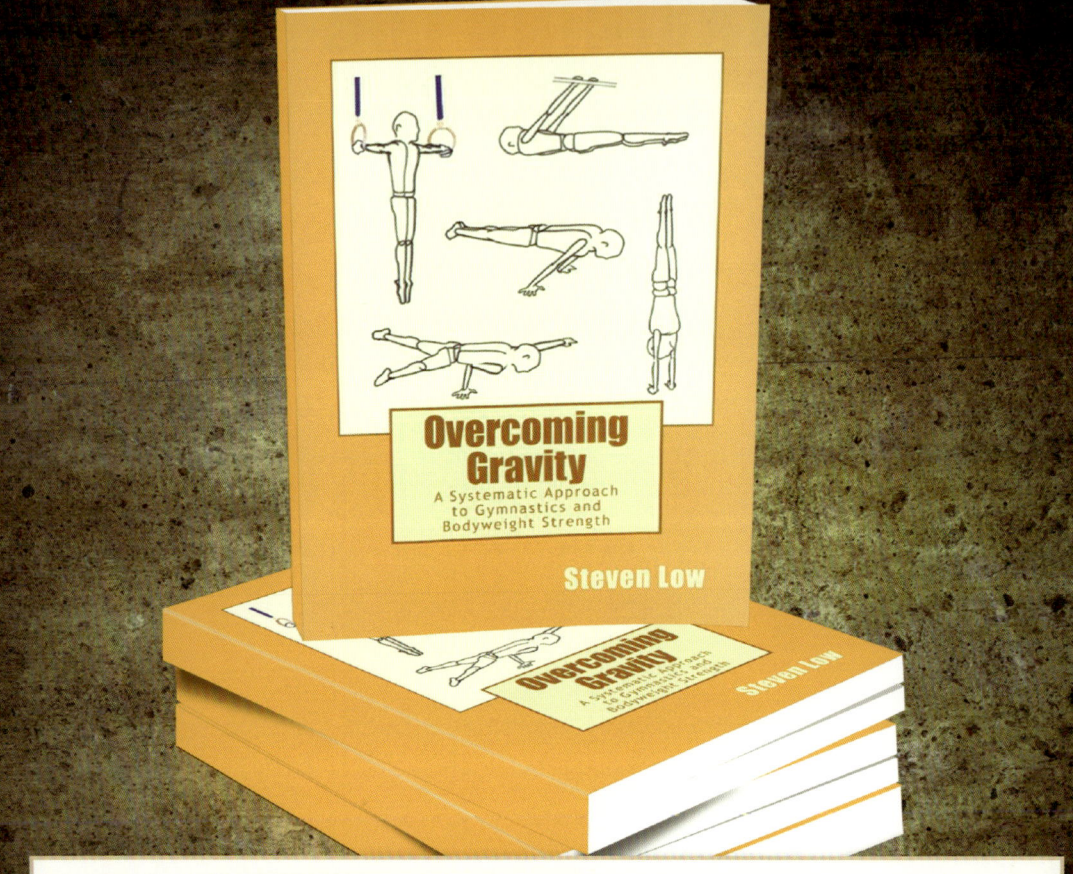

Great Bodyweight Strength Books # 5: Overcoming Gravity—Steven Low

Interested in discovering what gymnastics can teach you about strength and development? Look no further than this book. Huge (542 pages), comprehensive and loaded with scientific theory, Low's work is a masterpiece of bodyweight training. The book was written as a labor of love, not to make money. As soon as I got my hands on this manual I contacted Steve personally and told him that as a gymnastic-based calisthenics resource, his magnum opus would never be bettered.

CONVICT CONDITIONING — Ultimate Bodyweight TRAINING LOG

DAY: _____

DATE: _____

NO.	EXERCISE	SET 1	SET 2	SET 3	SET 4	SET 5

EXTRAS:

COMMENTS:

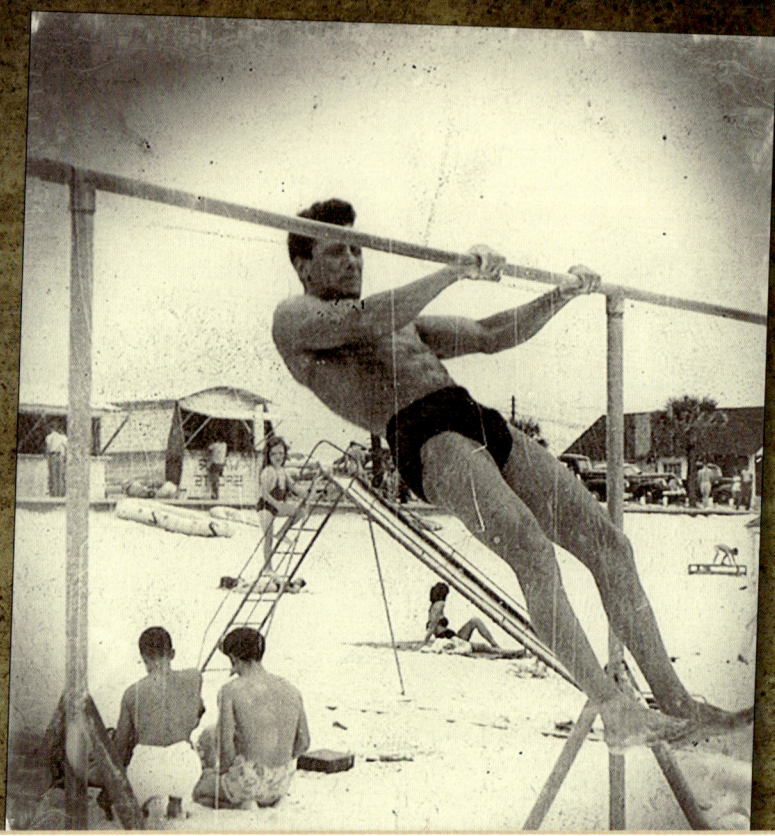

ON THE CTI:

Want to be as strong as the legendary Jasper Benincasa? Try his patented hold: the CTI. Get to the top of a pullup, then press your body away from the bar, arms straight. (TIP: it's called the *close-to-impossible* for a reason.)

PAUL "COACH" WADE'S CONVICT CONDITIONING ULTIMATE BODYWEIGHT TRAINING LOG

DAY: _____

DATE: _____

NO.	EXERCISE	SET 1	SET 2	SET 3	SET 4	SET 5

EXTRAS:

COMMENTS:

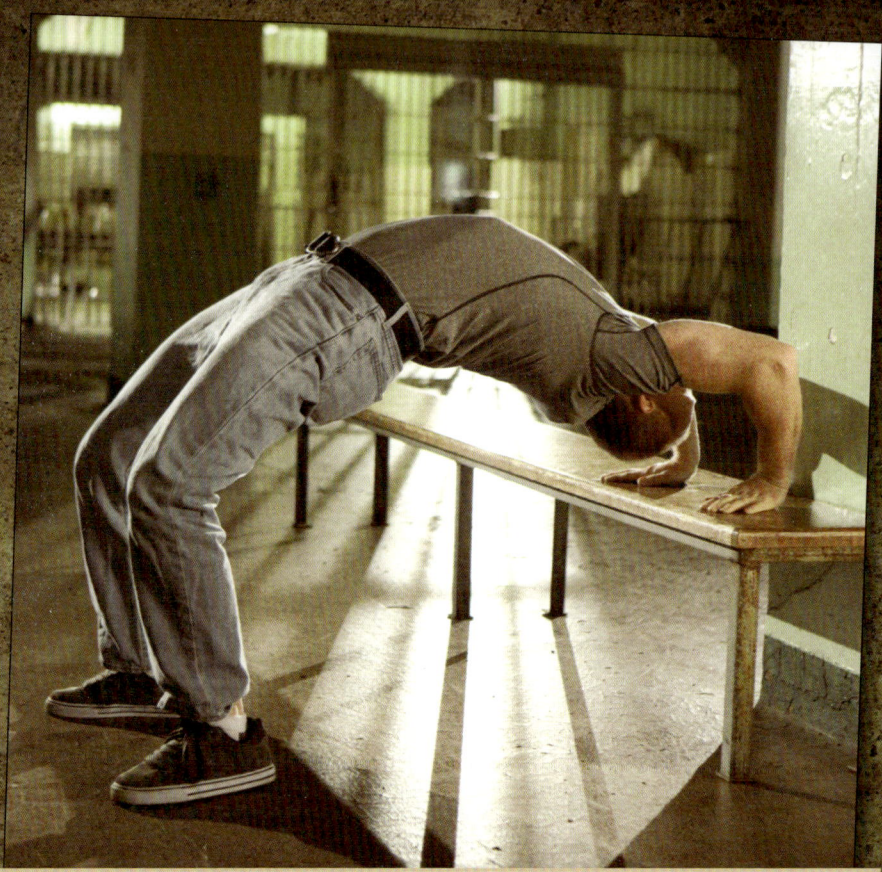

ON WEIGHT CONTROL:

One of the most powerful tools you have in improving your calisthenics performance isn't a training method at all—it's *weight control*. Calisthenics will burn lard from anyone's frame, but if you are 40, 50, or 60 pounds overweight, you will never get good at the exercises unless you show some discipline at the dinner table. Dropping weight isn't rocket science. Cut some junk, eat three squares a day, go to bed a little bit hungry and watch the weight fall off.

PAUL "COACH" WADE'S CONVICT CONDITIONING — Ultimate Bodyweight Training Log

DAY: _____

DATE: _____

NO.	EXERCISE	SET 1	SET 2	SET 3	SET 4	SET 5

EXTRAS:

COMMENTS:

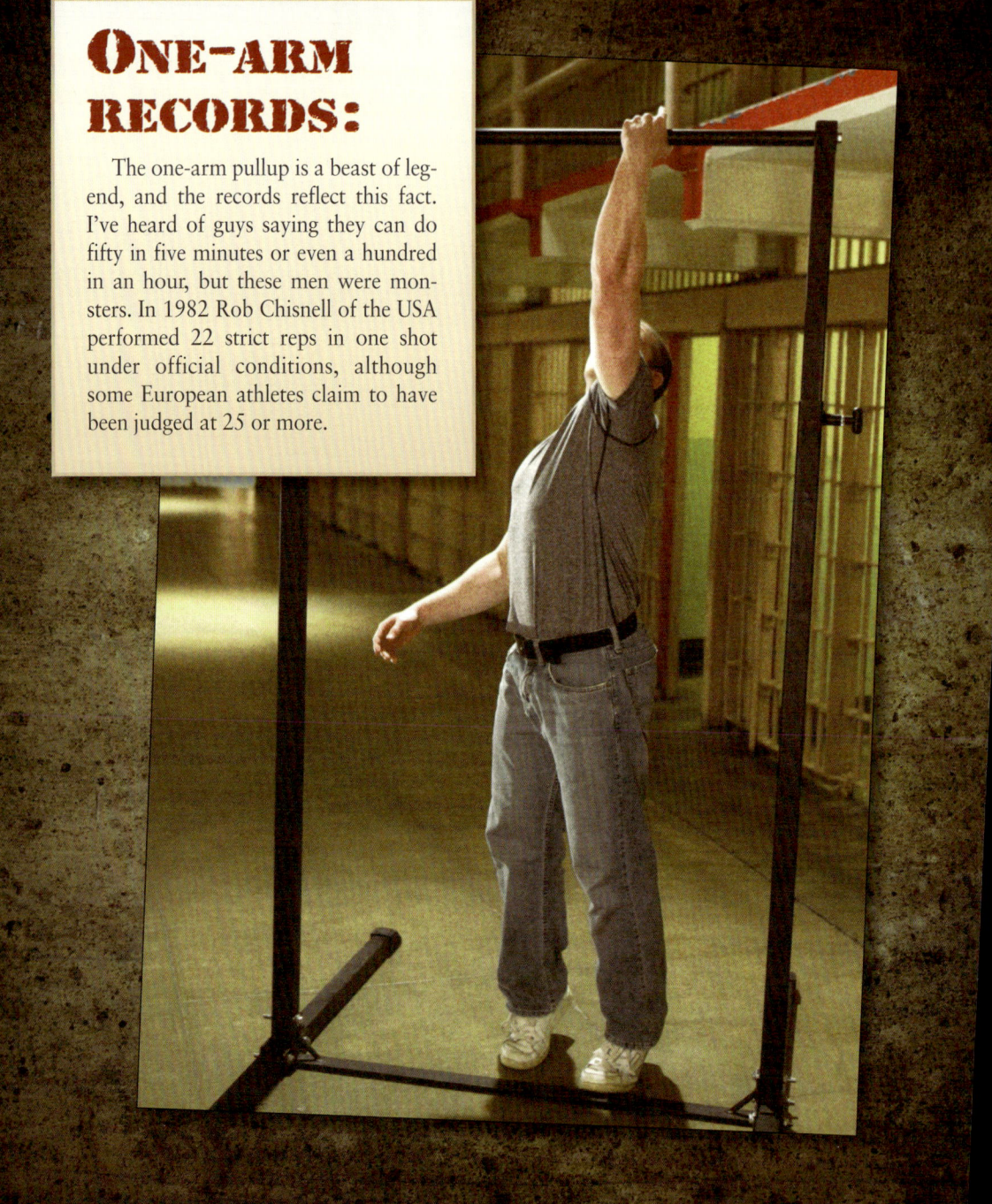

One-Arm Records:

The one-arm pullup is a beast of legend, and the records reflect this fact. I've heard of guys saying they can do fifty in five minutes or even a hundred in an hour, but these men were monsters. In 1982 Rob Chisnell of the USA performed 22 strict reps in one shot under official conditions, although some European athletes claim to have been judged at 25 or more.

CONVICT CONDITIONING — Ultimate Bodyweight Training Log

DAY: _____
DATE: _____

NO.	EXERCISE	SET 1	SET 2	SET 3	SET 4	SET 5

EXTRAS:

COMMENTS:

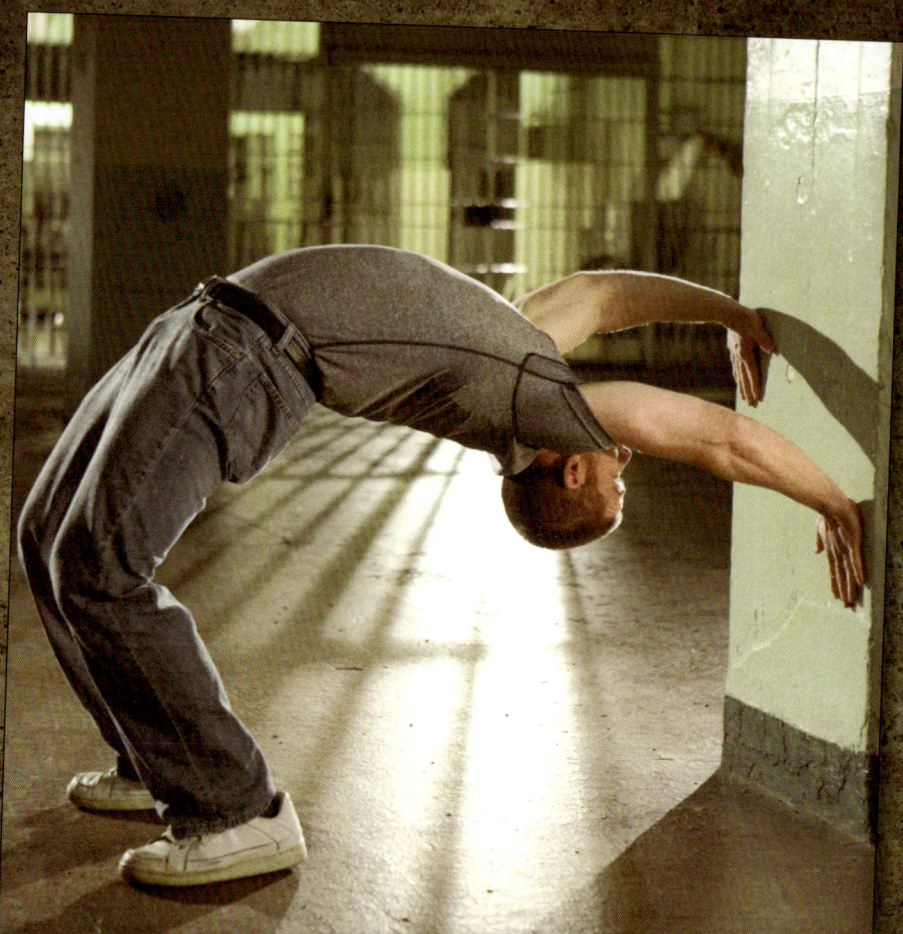

On "more is better":

Athletes training with barbells and dumbbells often get stuck in a "more is better" mindset—they get obsessed with adding more and more weight over time. Bodyweight athletes should steer clear of this attitude. Instead of asking how much *more* you can lift, begin thinking: *how can I use my body <u>better</u> every time I train?*

PAUL "COACH" WADE'S CONVICT CONDITIONING ULTIMATE BODYWEIGHT TRAINING LOG

DAY: _____

DATE: _____

NO.	EXERCISE	SET 1	SET 2	SET 3	SET 4	SET 5

EXTRAS:

COMMENTS:

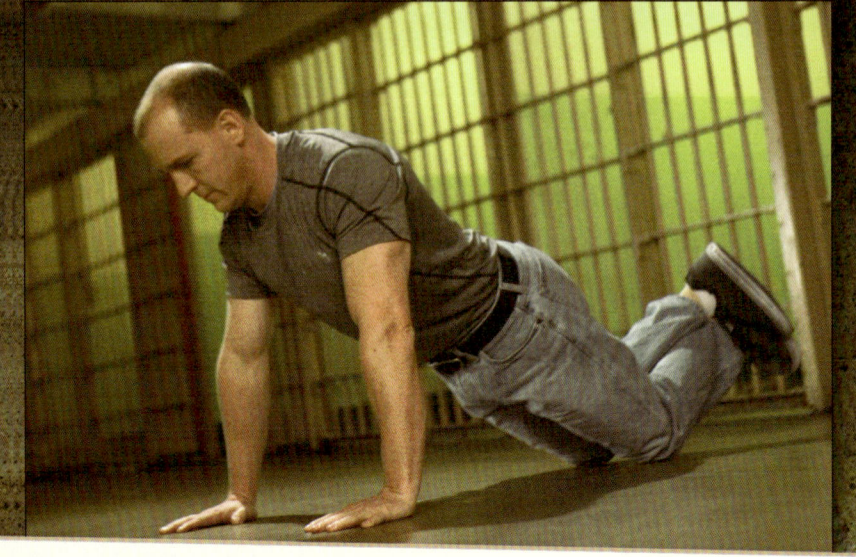

ON DROP SETS:

Bodybuilders who train with weights know all about "drop sets": they perform an exercise with a fixed weight, and when things get tough they drop the weight and keep on going—sometimes dropping the weight three or four times in a set. Fewer athletes realize that you can also apply this brutal method to bodyweight training: just hit your rep target, then move to an easier exercise. For example, if you finish a set of *close pushups*, you can immediately move to *full pushups* to get a few more reps; then *kneeling pushups*; and so on.

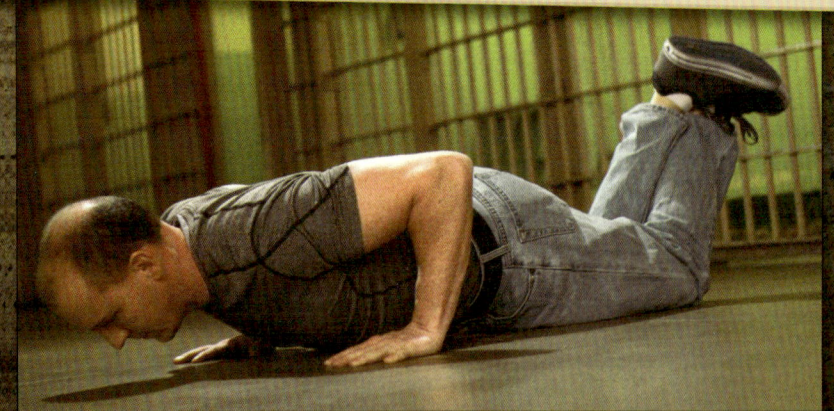

PAUL "COACH" WADE'S CONVICT CONDITIONING — Ultimate Bodyweight Training Log

DAY: _____
DATE: _____

NO.	EXERCISE	SET 1	SET 2	SET 3	SET 4	SET 5

EXTRAS:

COMMENTS:

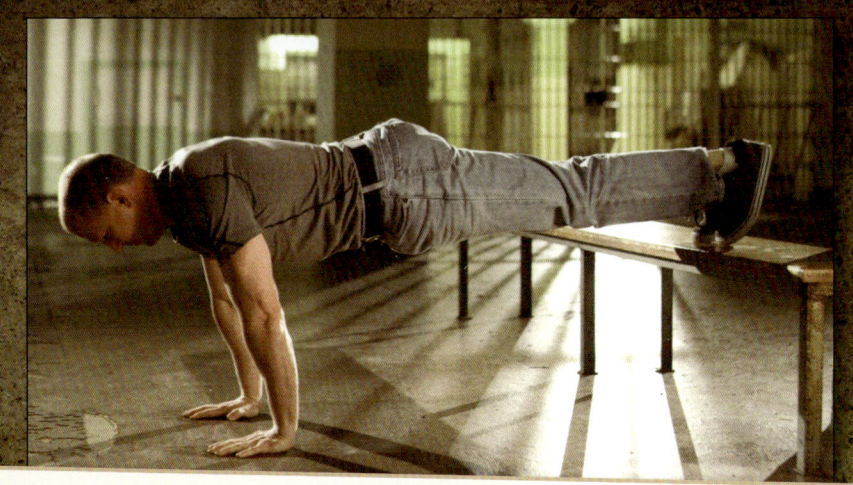

ON DECLINE PUSHUPS:

Somewhere in-between the *flat pushup* and the *handstand pushup* lies the *decline pushup*. These make for an excellent variant to work the anterior (front) deltoids and the upper pecs around the collarbone. Hitch your feet up on a secure object and lower your chin until it comes close to the floor before thrusting back up. Like most bodyweight exercises, declines can be performed progressively—keep putting your feet on higher objects over time.

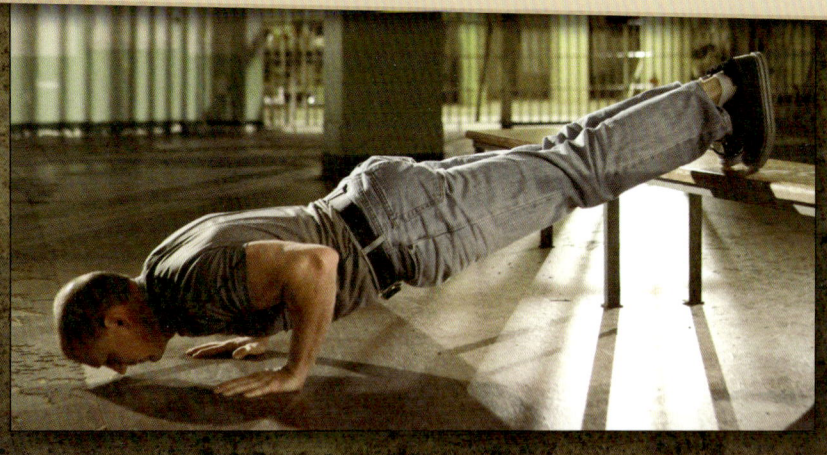

PAUL "COACH" WADE'S CONVICT CONDITIONING — Ultimate Bodyweight Training Log

DAY: _____

DATE: _____

NO.	EXERCISE	SET 1	SET 2	SET 3	SET 4	SET 5

EXTRAS:

COMMENTS:

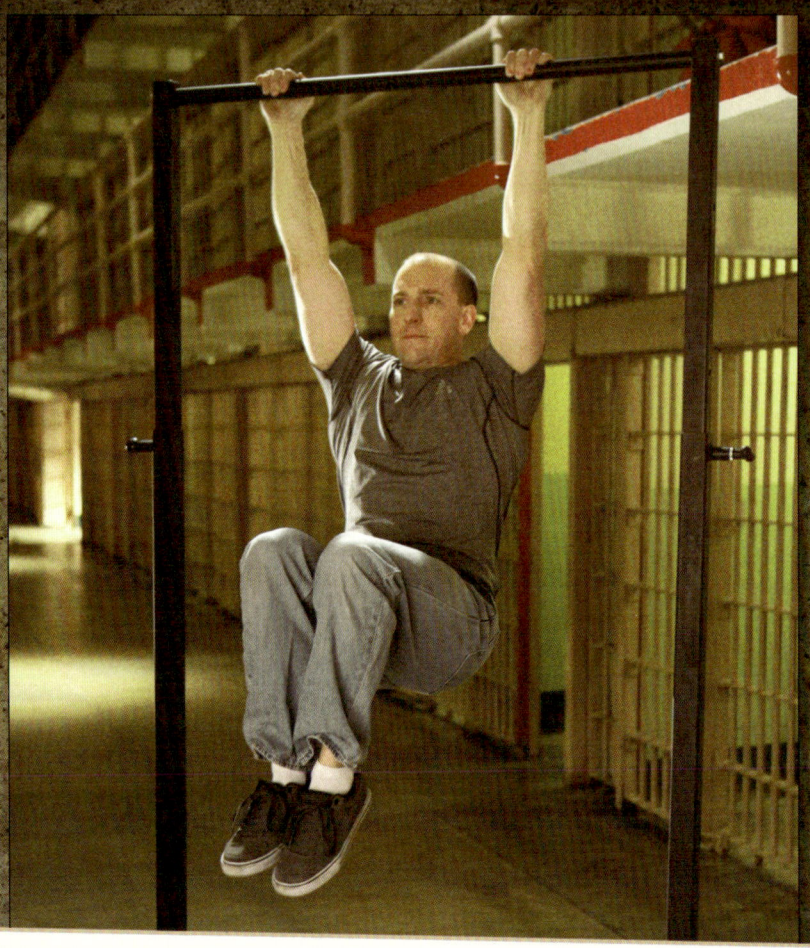

ON HANGING KNEE RAISES:

Coaches who sneer at simple hanging knee raises are really missing a trick. Human beings need to lift the knees when running, jumping or climbing (or even kneeing a mugger in the nuts). Raising the knees against gravity is a fundamental movement pattern and all athletes should spend a chunk of their career strengthening the muscles that get it done!

PAUL "COACH" WADE'S CONVICT CONDITIONING
ULTIMATE BODYWEIGHT TRAINING LOG

DAY: _____
DATE: _____

NO.	EXERCISE	SET 1	SET 2	SET 3	SET 4	SET 5

EXTRAS:

COMMENTS:

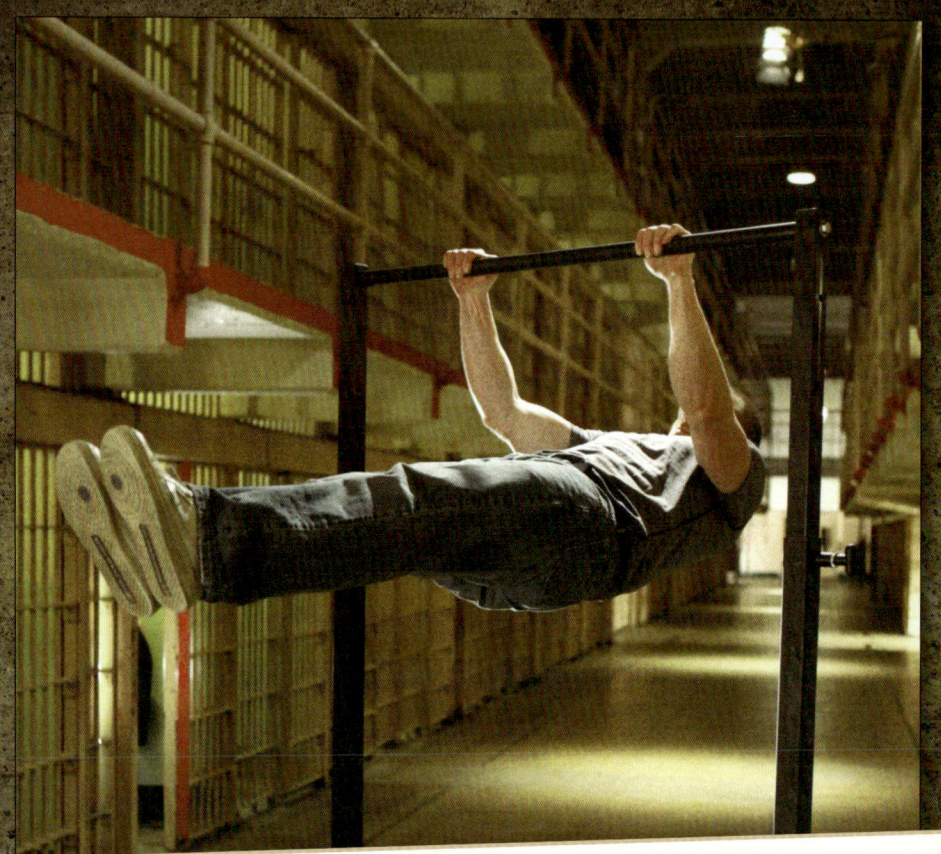

ON REVERSE PLANCHES:

What gymnasts call the *front lever* many convicts call the *reverse planche* or *reverse plank*. This is a powerful total-body static hold which builds huge strength in the upper back musculature. The full version of this exercise will be too tough for most experimenters, but you can work into it progressively. Begin with the legs bent and gradually increase leverage by extending just one leg; then straighten both legs, but spread wide apart. Over time, bring the legs in from the split position to form the Master Step.

PAUL "COACH" WADE'S CONVICT CONDITIONING

Ultimate Bodyweight Training Log

DAY: _____

DATE: _____

NO.	EXERCISE	SET 1	SET 2	SET 3	SET 4	SET 5

EXTRAS:

COMMENTS:

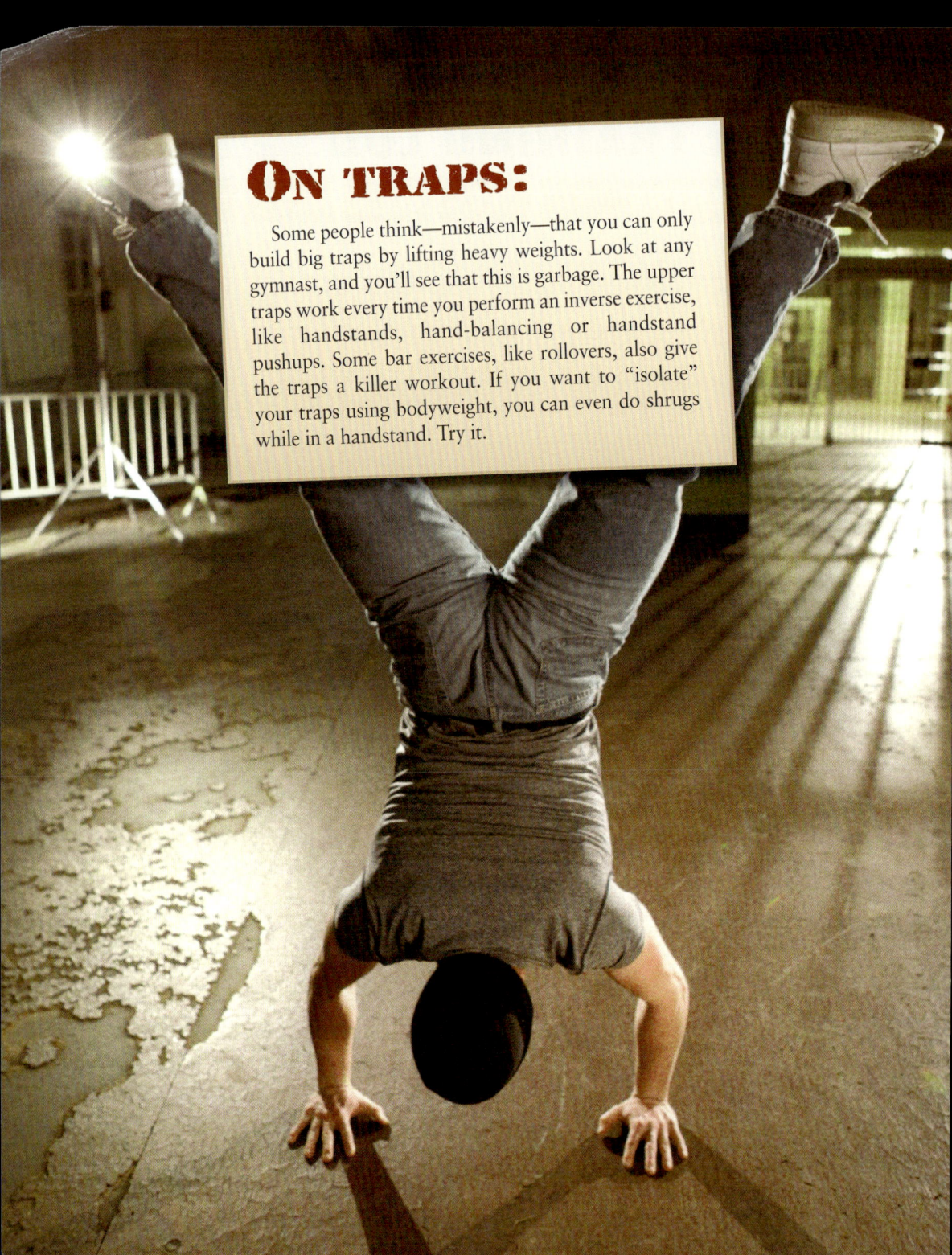

ON TRAPS:

Some people think—mistakenly—that you can only build big traps by lifting heavy weights. Look at any gymnast, and you'll see that this is garbage. The upper traps work every time you perform an inverse exercise, like handstands, hand-balancing or handstand pushups. Some bar exercises, like rollovers, also give the traps a killer workout. If you want to "isolate" your traps using bodyweight, you can even do shrugs while in a handstand. Try it.

CONVICT CONDITIONING: Ultimate Bodyweight Training Log

DAY: _____
DATE: _____

NO.	EXERCISE	SET 1	SET 2	SET 3	SET 4	SET 5

EXTRAS:

COMMENTS:

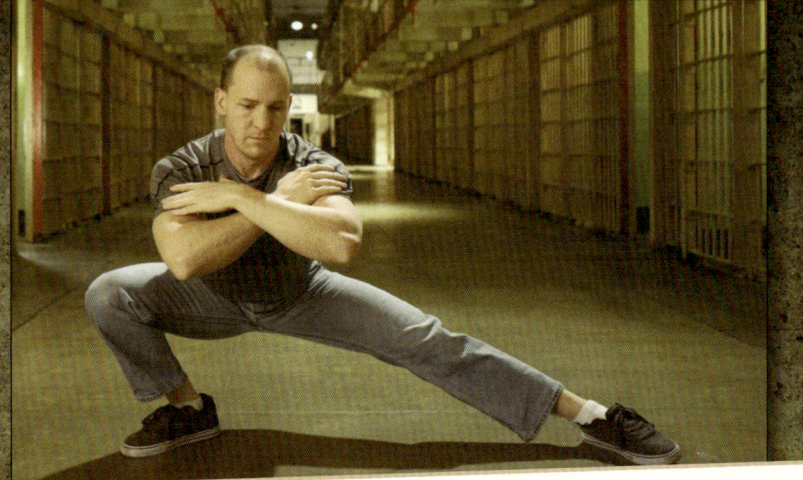

On side squats:

Most bodyweight athletes spend their leg workouts squatting straight *up-and-down*. What about squatting from *side-to-side*? Side squats improve strength in the hips, increase mobility and work the inner thigh muscles in a different way. You can perform them one leg at a time, but I prefer the moving version, alternating leg to leg. Focus on depth, great form and build your reps slowly.

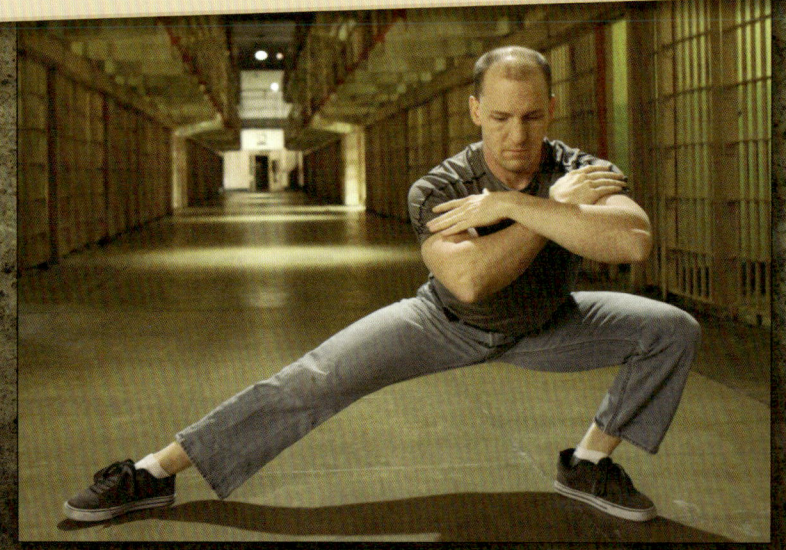

PAUL "COACH" WADE'S CONVICT CONDITIONING Ultimate Bodyweight TRAINING LOG

DAY: _____
DATE: _____

NO.	EXERCISE	SET 1	SET 2	SET 3	SET 4	SET 5

EXTRAS:

COMMENTS:

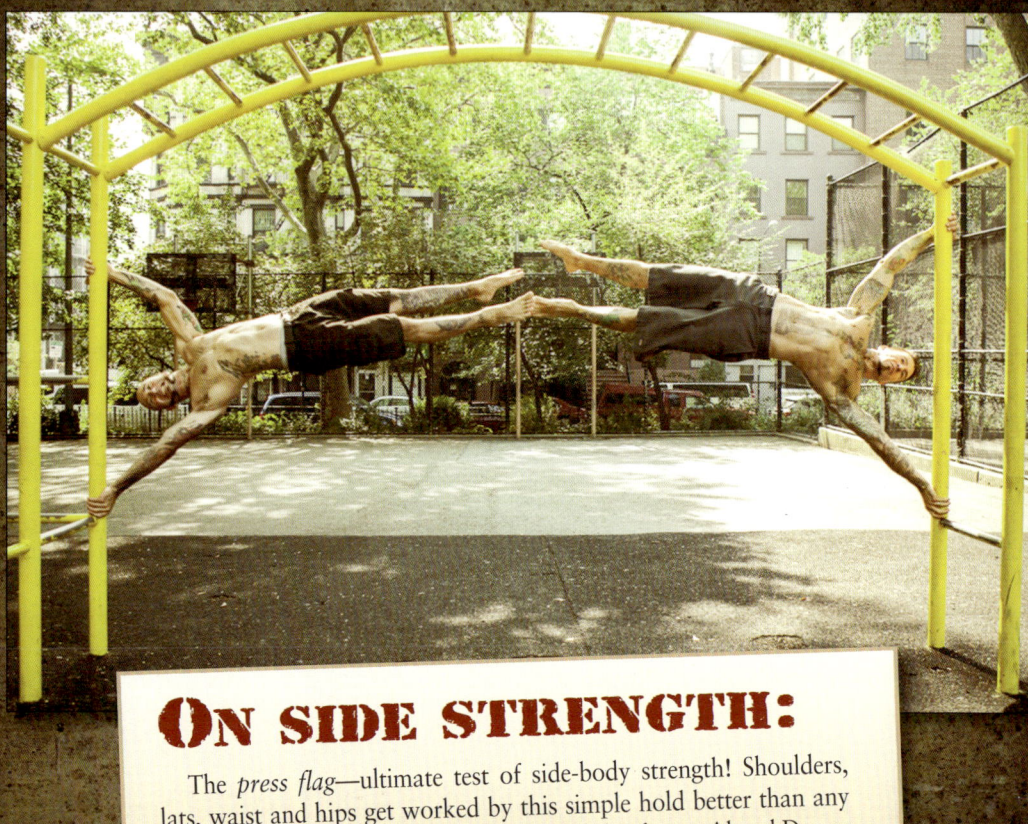

ON SIDE STRENGTH:

The *press flag*—ultimate test of side-body strength! Shoulders, lats, waist and hips get worked by this simple hold better than any million dollar machine designed by the minds of men. Al and Danny Kavadlo are masters of this hold—trust me, it ain't easy to smile while you're doing it!

PAUL "COACH" WADE'S CONVICT CONDITIONING ULTIMATE BODYWEIGHT TRAINING LOG

DAY: _____

DATE: _____

NO.	EXERCISE	SET 1	SET 2	SET 3	SET 4	SET 5

EXTRAS:

COMMENTS:

Sakamoto's HSPUs:

Most weight-lifters are burnt-out by their 30's, but calisthenics works *with* the body, and keeps you stronger for longer. At the youthful age of 52, Mako Sakamoto broke the world record with 163 unsupported handstand pushups—and these weren't down to his *head*, they were down to his *shoulders*. At sixty—and no longer training to break records—Sakamoto could "easily" perform 75 perfect reps!

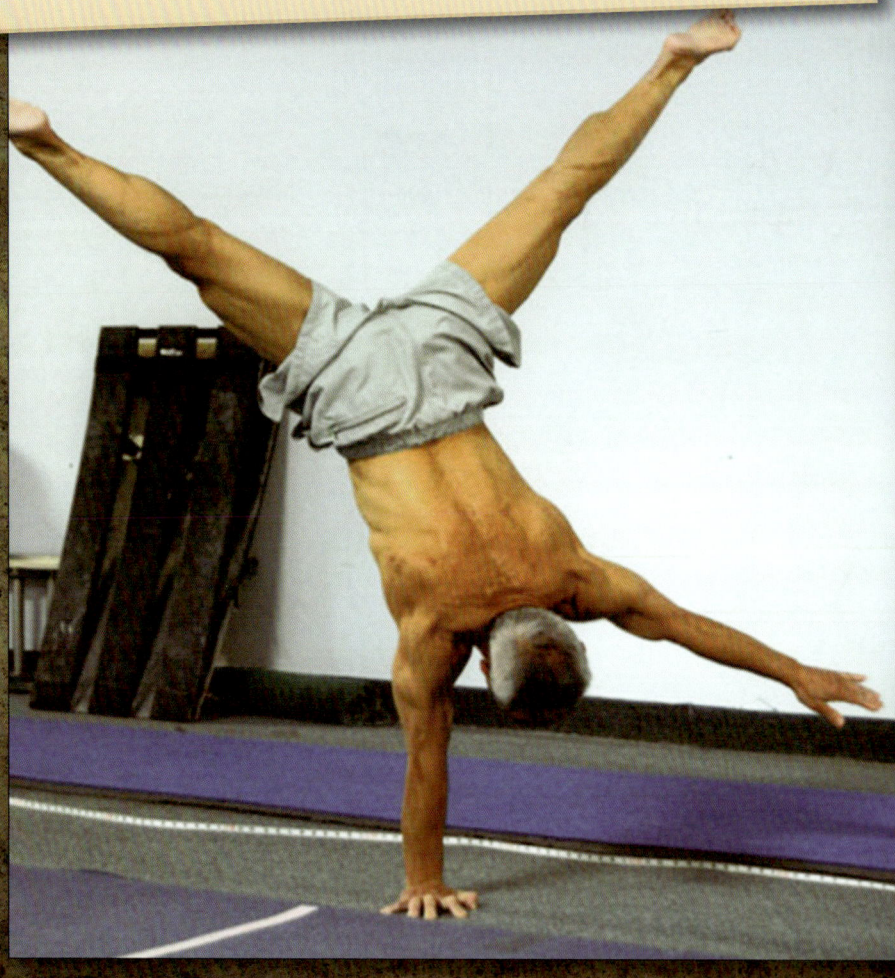

PAUL "COACH" WADE'S CONVICT CONDITIONING Ultimate Bodyweight TRAINING LOG

DAY: _____

DATE: _____

NO.	EXERCISE	SET 1	SET 2	SET 3	SET 4	SET 5

EXTRAS:

COMMENTS:

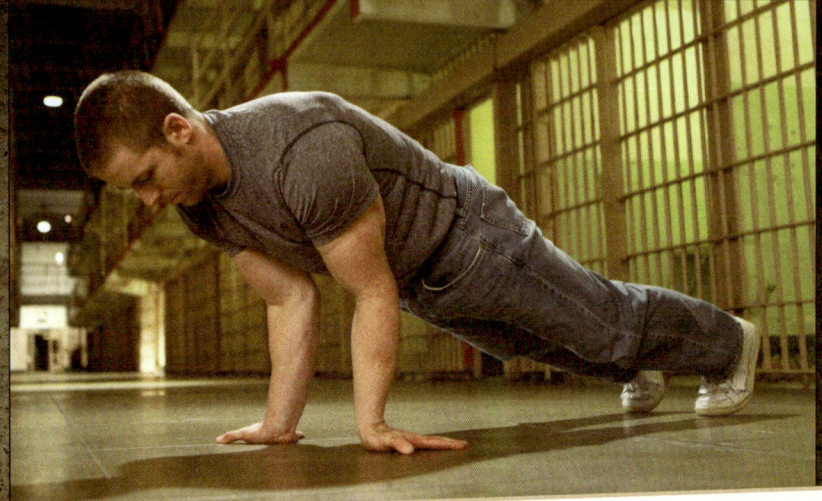

ON ELBOW LEVERS:

Elbow levers are a powerful total-body hold which radically strengthen the shoulders and arms. If you want to master this cool exercise, first make sure you are comfortable with the *crow stand* described in **Convict Conditioning**. From the crow stand position, there are several ways to extend your legs outwards behind you. As with so many bodyweight feats, the impossible becomes simple when you break it up into little chunks.

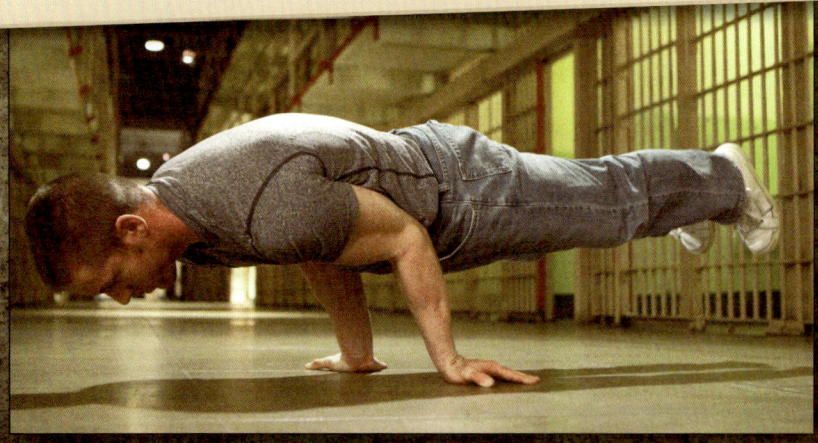

PAUL "COACH" WADE'S CONVICT CONDITIONING ULTIMATE BODYWEIGHT TRAINING LOG

DAY: _____
DATE: _____

NO.	EXERCISE	SET 1	SET 2	SET 3	SET 4	SET 5

EXTRAS:

COMMENTS:

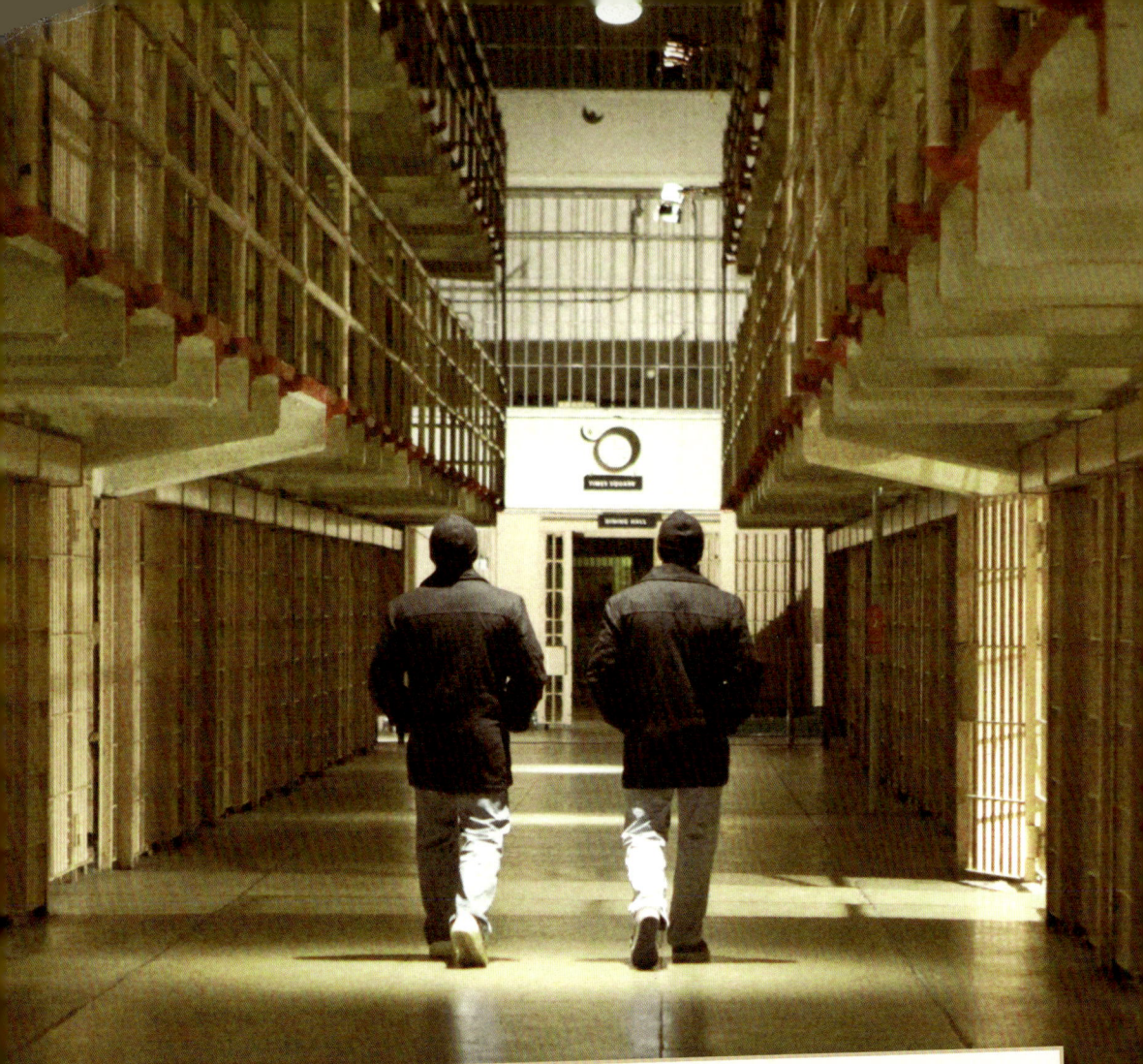

ON MOVING ON:

All "systems"—no matter how good—are ultimately prisons. They are confining for the mind and body. *Convict Conditioning* is no different. Spend time with the system, absorb what it has to teach. When the time comes for you to change your training, or develop further in a different direction, you must do so. There is no "dogma" in *Convict Conditioning*. Eventually all students will evolve beyond it, and build their own "system" to live in for a while.

PART III:
Charts & Checklists

Calisthenics Anatomy

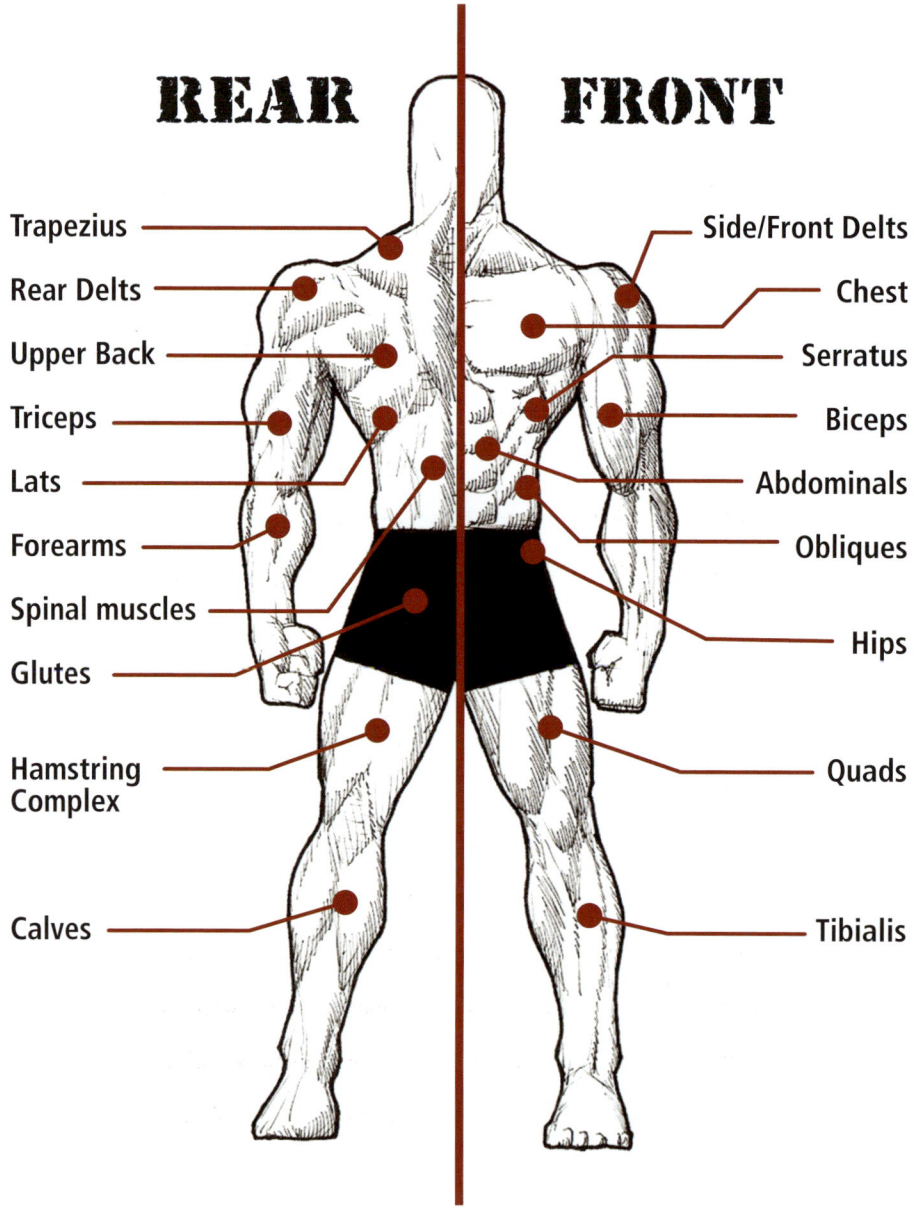

Calisthenics Anatomy

Muscle Groups:	Calisthenics Techniques:
Trapezius:	All handstand work
Side/front delts:	Handstands, handstand pushups, hand-balancing, pushups
Rear delts:	Horizontal pulls, pullups, bar pulls, front levers
Upper back:	Horizontal pulls, pullups, bar pulls, front levers
Chest:	Pushups, dips, sentry pullups, crawling drills, deep breathing techniques
Lats:	All pullups (jackknife, close, clapping, etc.)
Serratus:	Pushups, dips, leg raises, pullups
Biceps:	Pullups, close pullups, elbow levers
Triceps:	Handstand work, all pushups, dips, bodyweight extensions
Forearms:	Pullups, bar and towel hangs, fingertip pushups
Spinal muscles:	All bridges, hyperextensions, squats
Abdominals:	Leg raises, sit-ups, kip-ups, L-holds
Obliques:	Flag work, twisting leg raises, spinal twists
Glutes:	Bridging, squats, hyperextensions, sprinting
Front hips:	Leg raises, L-holds, sit-ups, kip-ups, spinal twists
Quads:	All squats, plyometric jumps, sprints, hill sprints
Hamstrings:	Bridges, straight bridges, squats, all jumps, sprints
Calves:	Calf raises, squatting calf raises, all jumps, sprints
Tibialis:	One-leg squats, inverse bar hangs, ankle rolling

Personal Records

While you work your way through the daily log entries—workout by workout—you will naturally reach a handful of high points in your training. These may be planned; they may even take you by surprise. These high points are what coaches call PRs: *Personal Records*. When you feel proud of what you've achieved in your training, it's a positive act to note your achievement down. That's what this section is for.

Personal Records are just that—personal. What's cool and impressive to you doesn't need to be cool and impressive to anybody else in the universe. Remember that while you note your PRs down. Remember also that PRs needn't be back-breaking or standardized for competition—they can relate to *any* area of physical culture. For example:

- Achieving a peak amount of reps on an exercise
- Moving up to an exercise you didn't think you could perform
- Meeting a training goal (page 7)
- Any workout where you finally mastered a technique, or had a breakthrough in your training style
- An increase in muscle size (e.g., arm size)
- Fat loss/waist reduction
- Any set where you attained a high mental level ("the zone" baby!)
- Overcoming a previous weakness (e.g., getting stronger legs)

All these accomplishments are worthy of recording for posterity. So do it!

Personal Records

DATE	ACCOMPLISHMENT

Six Month Weight Stats

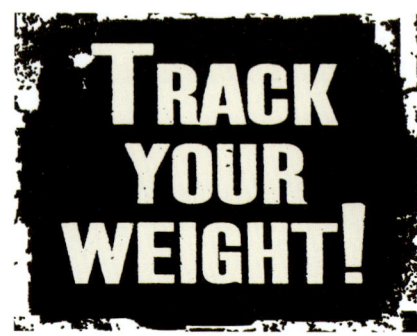

Health aside, every serious calisthenics athlete should keep track of their bodyweight for two reasons. The first reason is simple *performance awareness*. A weight-lifter wouldn't try to lift a barbell without knowing its weight, right? But in calisthenics, your body is your barbell. You need to know how much it weighs, otherwise it's tough to gauge your progress over time. Let's say six months ago you could do six strict pullups, but your reps haven't gone up in that time. Most people would assume that they haven't made any progress. But what if you had put on 20 lbs during that period? You'd be lifting 20lbs more for the same amount of reps—so you would have made progress, but this would be impossible to realize unless you kept track of your weight on a regular basis.

The second reason has to do with *training efficiency*. If you want to continually move to harder and harder calisthenics exercises—one-arm pushups or one-leg squats, for example—you'll need to drop as much excess flab as possible. This is much easier to do if you keep track of your weight over time.

In the box below, write your current weight and your ideal training weight. It's a good rule of thumb for most athletes to weigh themselves weekly. On the opposite page, fill in the results.

DATE	CURRENT WEIGHT	IDEAL WEIGHT

Six Month Weight Stats

DATE	WEIGHT	DATE	WEIGHT

An obese ex-Marine once asked me for the best program he could use to improve his sub-par pullup performance. I told him that the best program he could follow over the next six months would be a good *nutritional* program—if he dropped fifty pounds, his pullups would become a damn sight easier!

Convict Conditioning: Pushup Table

STEP	TECHNIQUE	BEGINNER STANDARD	INTERMEDIATE STANDARD	PROGRESSION STANDARD
1	Wall Pushups	1 set of 10	2 sets of 25	3 sets of 50
2	Incline Pushups	1 set of 10	2 sets of 20	3 sets of 40
3	Kneeling Pushups	1 set of 10	2 sets of 15	3 sets of 30
4	Half Pushups	1 set of 8	2 sets of 12	2 sets of 25
5	Full Pushups	1 set of 5	2 sets of 10	2 sets of 20
6	Close Pushups	1 set of 5	2 sets of 10	2 sets of 20
7	Uneven Pushups	1 set of 5	2 sets of 10	2 sets of 20
8	½ One-Arm Pushups	1 set of 5	2 sets of 10	2 sets of 20
9	Lever Pushups	1 set of 5	2 sets of 10	2 sets of 20
10	One-Arm Pushups	1 set of 5	2 sets of 10	—

Convict Conditioning: Squat Table

STEP	TECHNIQUE	BEGINNER STANDARD	INTERMEDIATE STANDARD	PROGRESSION STANDARD
1	Shoulderstand Squats	1 set of 10	2 sets of 25	3 sets of 50
2	Jackknife Squats	1 set of 10	2 sets of 20	3 sets of 40
3	Supported Squats	1 set of 10	2 sets of 15	3 sets of 30
4	Half Squats	1 set of 8	2 sets of 35	2 sets of 50
5	Full Squats	1 set of 5	2 sets of 10	2 sets of 30
6	Close Squats	1 set of 5	2 sets of 10	2 sets of 20
7	Uneven Squats	1 set of 5	2 sets of 10	2 sets of 20
8	½ One-Leg Squats	1 set of 5	2 sets of 10	2 sets of 20
9	Assisted One-Leg Squats	1 set of 5	2 sets of 10	2 sets of 20
10	One-Leg Squats	1 set of 5	2 sets of 10	—

Convict Conditioning: Pullup Table

STEP	TECHNIQUE	BEGINNER STANDARD	INTERMEDIATE STANDARD	PROGRESSION STANDARD
1	Vertical Pulls	1 set of 10	2 sets of 20	3 sets of 40
2	Horizontal Pulls	1 set of 10	2 sets of 20	3 sets of 30
3	Jackknife Pulls	1 set of 10	2 sets of 15	3 sets of 20
4	Half Pullups	1 set of 8	2 sets of 11	2 sets of 15
5	Full Pullups	1 set of 5	2 sets of 8	2 sets of 10
6	Close Pullups	1 set of 5	2 sets of 8	2 sets of 10
7	Uneven Pullups	1 set of 5	2 sets of 7	2 sets of 9
8	½ One-Arm Pullups	1 set of 4	2 sets of 6	2 sets of 8
9	Assisted One-Arm Pullups	1 set of 3	2 sets of 5	2 sets of 7
10	One-Arm Pullups	1 set of 1	2 sets of 3	—

Convict Conditioning: Leg Raise Table

STEP	TECHNIQUE	BEGINNER STANDARD	INTERMEDIATE STANDARD	PROGRESSION STANDARD
1	Knee Tucks	1 set of 10	2 sets of 25	3 sets of 40
2	Flat Knee Raises	1 set of 10	2 sets of 20	3 sets of 35
3	Flat Bent Leg Raises	1 set of 10	2 sets of 15	3 sets of 30
4	Flat Frog Raises	1 set of 8	2 sets of 15	3 sets of 25
5	Flat Straight Leg Raises	1 set of 5	2 sets of 10	2 sets of 20
6	Hanging Knee Raises	1 set of 5	2 sets of 10	2 sets of 15
7	Hanging Bent Leg Raises	1 set of 5	2 sets of 10	2 sets of 15
8	Hanging Frog Raises	1 set of 5	2 sets of 10	2 sets of 15
9	Partial Leg Raises	1 set of 5	2 sets of 10	2 sets of 15
10	Hanging Leg Raises	1 set of 5	2 sets of 10	—

Convict Conditioning: Bridge Table

STEP	TECHNIQUE	BEGINNER STANDARD	INTERMEDIATE STANDARD	PROGRESSION STANDARD
1	Short Bridges	1 set of 10	2 sets of 25	3 sets of 50
2	Straight Bridges	1 set of 10	2 sets of 20	3 sets of 40
3	Angled Bridges	1 set of 8	2 sets of 15	3 sets of 30
4	Head Bridges	1 set of 8	2 sets of 15	2 sets of 25
5	Half Bridges	1 set of 8	2 sets of 15	2 sets of 20
6	Full Bridges	1 set of 6	2 sets of 10	2 sets of 15
7	Wall Walking Bridges (Down)	1 set of 3	2 sets of 6	2 sets of 10
8	Wall Walking Bridges (Up)	1 set of 2	2 sets of 4	2 sets of 8
9	Closing Bridges	1 set of 1	2 sets of 3	2 sets of 6
10	Stand-To-Stand Bridges	1 set of 1	2 sets of 3	—

Convict Conditioning: HSPU Table

STEP	TECHNIQUE	BEGINNER STANDARD	INTERMEDIATE STANDARD	PROGRESSION STANDARD
1	Wall Headstands	30 Seconds	1 Minute	2 Minutes
2	Crow Stands	10 Seconds	30 Seconds	1 Minute
3	Wall Handstands	30 Seconds	1 Minute	2 Minutes
4	½ Handstand Pushups	1 set of 5	2 sets of 10	2 sets of 20
5	Handstand Pushups	1 set of 5	2 sets of 10	2 sets of 15
6	Close HSPUs	1 set of 5	2 sets of 9	2 sets of 12
7	Uneven HSPUs	1 set of 5	2 sets of 8	2 sets of 10
8	½ One-Arm HSPUs	1 set of 4	2 sets of 6	2 sets of 8
9	Lever HSPUs	1 set of 3	2 sets of 4	2 sets of 6
10	One-Arm HSPUs	1 set of 1	2 sets of 2	—

NOTES: THESE END PAGES HAVE BEEN PURPOSELY LEFT BLANK

NOTES: These end pages have been Purposely left blank

NOTES: THESE END PAGES HAVE BEEN PURPOSELY LEFT BLANK

NOTES: THESE END PAGES HAVE BEEN PURPOSELY LEFT BLANK

NOTES: THESE END PAGES HAVE BEEN PURPOSELY LEFT BLANK

NOTES: THESE END PAGES HAVE BEEN PURPOSELY LEFT BLANK

NOTES: THESE END PAGES HAVE BEEN PURPOSELY LEFT BLANK

NOTES: THESE END PAGES HAVE BEEN PURPOSELY LEFT BLANK

The athletes who modeled for the photos in this book were Max Shank (left) and Brett Jones (right) who both endured several brutal days of training incarcerated at Alcatraz with inhuman stamina and good grace. Thank you, gentlemen: you kick ass.

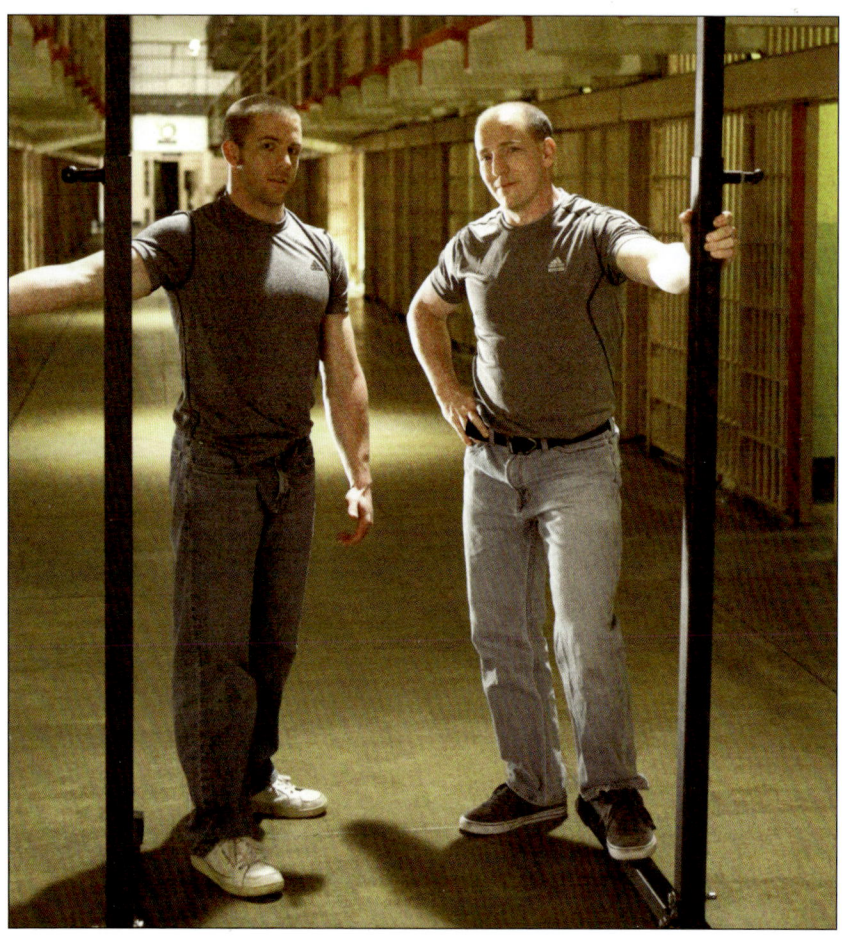

A massive thanks must also go to the great John Du Cane. The Alcatraz shoot was his brainchild, and without it this book would have been impossible.

The photographer was the amazing Marc Blondin. I think Marc's great work speaks for itself: *incredible*.

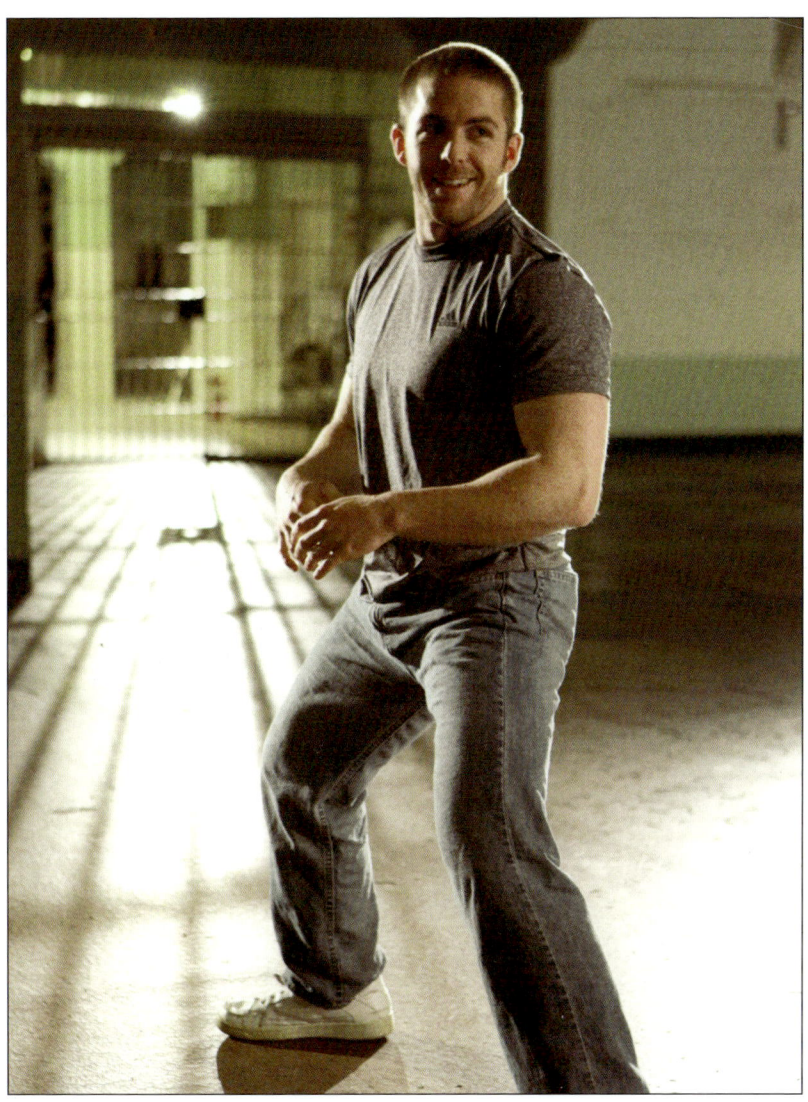

Max Shank is a strength coach, RKC instructor, and corrective exercise specialist based in Encinitas, CA. As well as being a highly talented bodyweight athlete, Max is also a martial artist who has competed in the Highland Games. Max is the owner of Ambition Athletics and can be reached through his website at: *www.ambitionathletics.com*.

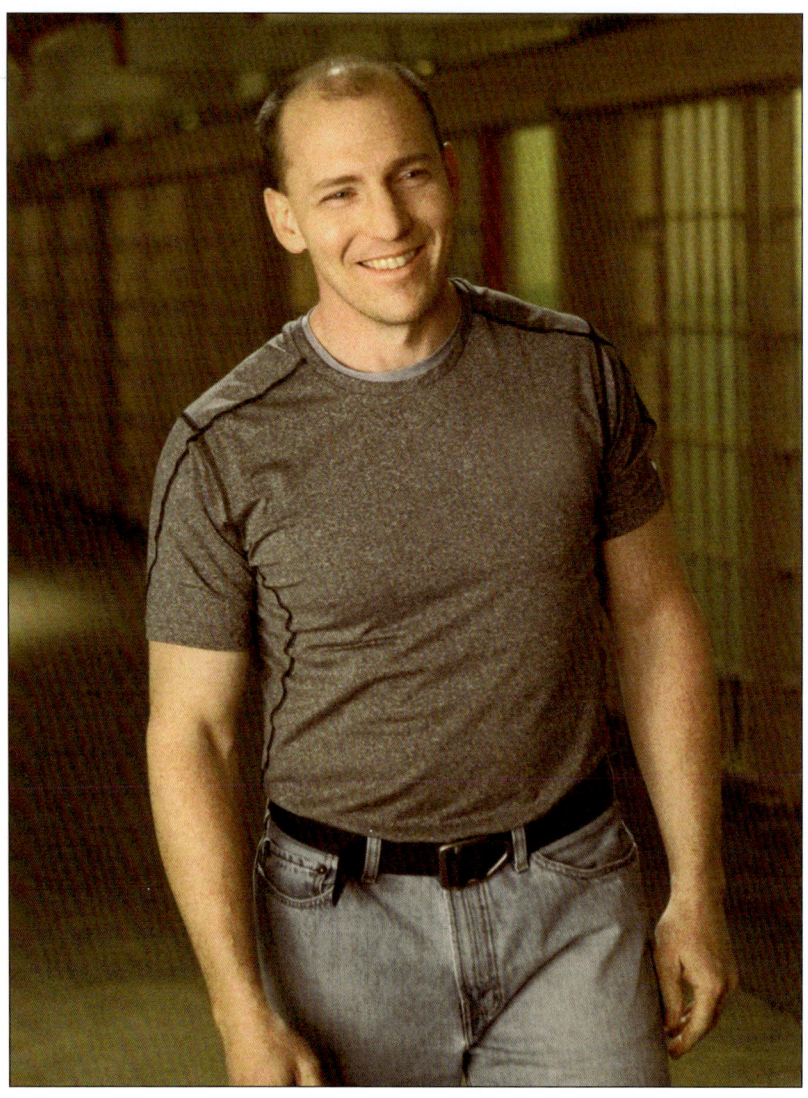

Brett Jones is one of the most highly respected strength and movement coaches in the world. As well as being a Master RKC, CK-FMS and a Certified Indian Club specialist, Brett is also incredibly knowledgeable in the field of strength calisthenics, and was the original editor of Convict Conditioning. Find him at ***www.appliedstrength.com***.

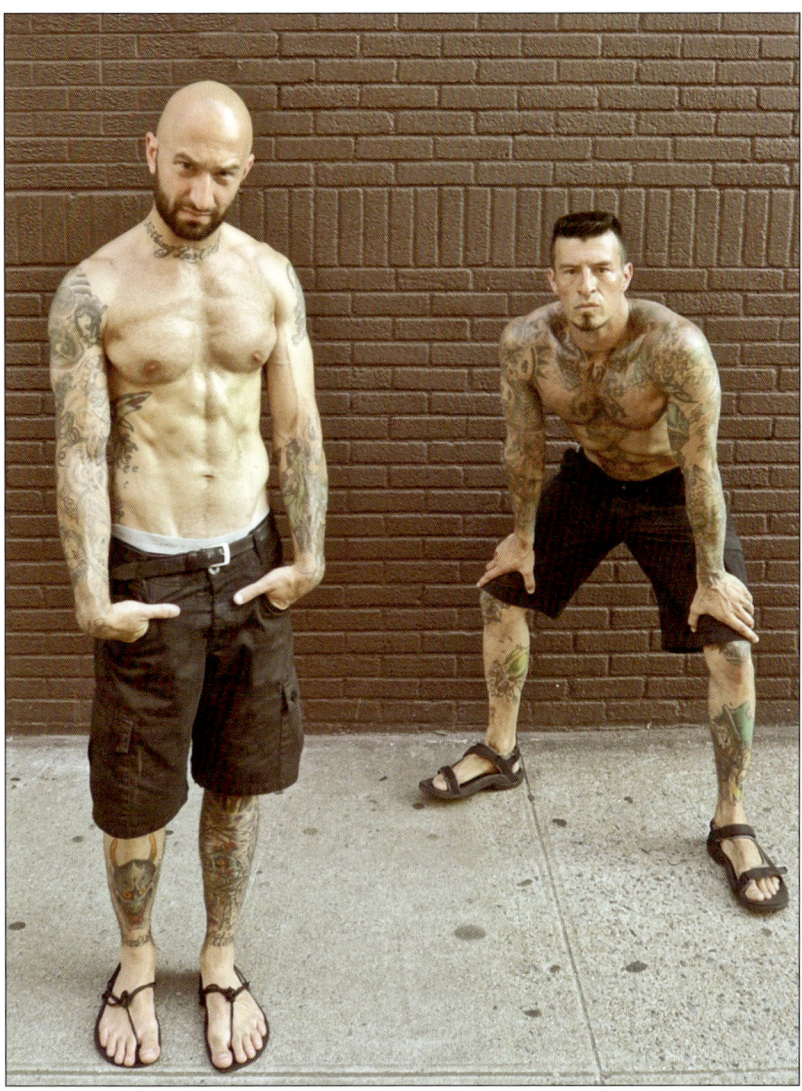

Al and Danny Kavadlo are brothers living and training in New York City. Nobody does calisthenics quite like these guys, and as a result they have become two of the most successful and sought-after trainers in America today. Al can be found at ***www.AlKavadlo.com***, and Danny can be reached through ***www.DannyTheTrainer.com***.

Extra Acknowledgements

The shots of Al and his brother, Danny, were graciously donated by the lean, serene, muscle-up machine himself. Many of these shots have never been seen anywhere else. The shots on pages 66, 100, 174 and 271 were taken by Colleen Leung, and the beautiful partner training images of Al with Danny on pages 36 and 240 were taken by Trevor Reid. Fine work!

It was an honor and a pleasure to include the incredible Makoto Sakamoto in this book. My heartfelt thanks go to Dr Max Vercruyssen for his great stories, and for putting me in touch with Makoto Sensei, and I want to thank Mako Sensei for giving me permission to include the shot on page 242. The Hawaaii Academy is clearly doing something very right to have these men on board! Check out their site at: *www.hawaiiacademy.com*.

I also want to extend my thanks to Logan Christopher, who was kind enough to donate a very cool photo of himself to this project. Logan can be found at *www.legendarystrength.com*, but you should definitely also visit his site *www.lostartofhandbalancing.com*, which is full of ice cold resources and ideas—really the major hub for handbalancing and wannabe balancers. You cannot put a foot wrong if you follow any of Logan's bodyweight training advice.

The image of Brook's Kubik's book is drawn from his Dino training website. Pick up a copy of the book here: *www.brookskubik.com/dinosaur_bodyweight.html*.

Last but definitely not least, a massive thank you needs to Big D, Derek Brigham, genius designer who has saved my ass on this project what seems like a million times. Thanks for not putting a hit out on me yet, my man. *www.dbrigham.com*.

Now…why the hell are you still reading this crap? Order another training logbook and do some more pushups!

How Do YOU Stack Up Against These 6 Signs of a TRUE Physical Specimen?

According to Paul Wade's Convict Conditioning you earn the right to call yourself a "true physical specimen" if you can perform the following:

✓ 1. AT LEAST one set of 5 one-arm pushups each side— with the ELITE goal of 100 sets each side

✓ 2. AT LEAST one set of 5 one-leg squats each side— with the ELITE goal of 2 sets of 50 each side

✓ 3. AT LEAST one set of 1 one-arm pullups each side— with the ELITE goal of 2 sets of 6 each side

✓ 4. AT LEAST one set of 5 hanging straight leg raises— with the ELITE goal of 2 sets of 30

✓ 5. AT LEAST one set of 1 stand-to-stand bridges— with the ELITE goal of 2 sets of 30

✓ 6. AT LEAST one set of 1 one-arm handstand pushups— with the ELITE goal of 1 set of 5

Well, how DO you stack up?

Convict Conditioning
*How to Bust Free of All Weakness—
Using the Lost Secrets of Supreme
Survival Strength*
By Paul "Coach" Wade   #B41 $39.95
Paperback 8.5 x 11   320 pages
191 photos, charts and illustrations

www.dragondoor.com
1·800·899·5111

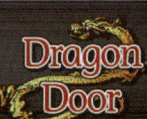

Order *Convict Conditioning* online:
www.dragondoor.com/B41

If you liked Paul "Coach" Wade's *Convict Conditioning* books, we recommend you visit www.dragondoor.com for information on related fitness resources.

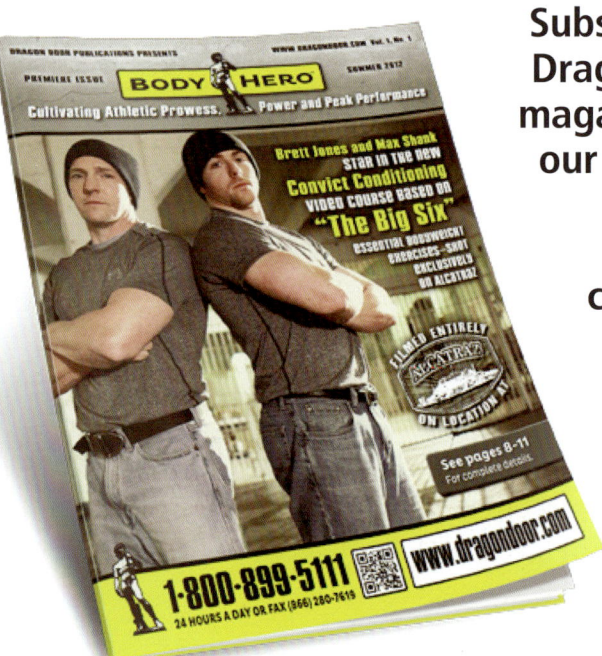

Subscribe at no charge to Dragon Door's Body Hero magazine and consult with our many experts on the dragondoor.com strength and conditioning forum

Order online or call
1-800-899-5111

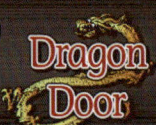

www.dragondoor.com

Chances are that whatever athletic level you have achieved, there are some serious gaps in your OVERALL strength program. Gaps that stop you short of being able to claim status as a truly accomplished strength athlete.

The good news is that—in *Convict Conditioning*—**Paul Wade** has laid out a brilliant 6-set system of 10 progressions which allows you to master these elite levels.

And you could be starting at almost any age and in almost in any condition…

Paul Wade has given you the keys—ALL the keys you'll ever need— that will open door, after door, after door for you in your quest for supreme physical excellence. Yes, it will be the hardest work you'll ever have to do. And yes, 97% of those who pick up **Convict Conditioning**, frankly, won't have the guts and the fortitude to make it. But if you make it even half-way through **Paul's Progressions**, you'll be stronger than almost anyone you encounter. Ever.

Dragon Door Customer Acclaim for Paul Wade's Convict Conditioning

A Strength Training Guide That Will Never Be Duplicated!

"I knew within the first chapter of reading this book that I was in for something special and unique. The last time I felt this same feeling was when reading *Power to the People!* To me this is the Body Weight equivalent to Pavel's masterpiece.

Books like this can never be duplicated. Paul Wade went through a unique set of circumstances of doing time in prison with an 'old time' master of calisthenics. Paul took these lessons from this 70 year old strong man and mastered them over a period of 20 years while 'doing time'. He then taught these methods to countless prisoners and honed his teaching to perfection.

I believe that extreme circumstances like this are what it takes to create a true masterpiece. I know that 'masterpiece' is a strong word, but this is as close as it gets. No other body weight book I have read (and I have a huge fitness library)…comes close to this as far as gaining incredible strength from body weight exercise.

Just like Power to the People, I am sure I will read this over and over again…mastering the principles that Paul Wade took 20 years to master.

Outstanding Book!"

—*Rusty Moore - Fitness Black Book - Seattle, WA*

I've packed all of my other training books away!

"I read CC in one go. I couldn't put it down. I have purchased a lot of bodyweight training books in the past, and have always been pretty disappointed. They all seem to just have pictures of different exercises, and no plan whatsoever on how to implement them and progress with them. But not with this one. The information in this book is AWESOME! I like to have a clear, logical plan of progression to follow, and that is what this book gives. I have put all of my other training books away. CC is the only system I am going to follow. This is now my favorite training book ever!"

—*Lyndan - Australia*

This book sets the standard, ladies and gentlemen

"It's difficult to describe just how much this book means to me. I've been training hard since I was in the RAF nearly ten years ago, and to say this book is a breakthrough is an understatement. How often do you really read something so new, so fresh? This book contains a complete new system of calisthenics drawn from American prison training methods. When I say 'system' I mean it. It's complete (rank beginner to expert), it's comprehensive (all the exercises and photos are here), it's graded (progressions from exercise to exercise are smooth and pre-determined) and it's totally original."

—Andy McMann - Ponty, Wales, GB

Convict Conditioning
How to Bust Free of All Weakness— Using the Lost Secrets of Supreme Survival Strength
By Paul "Coach" Wade #B41 $39.95

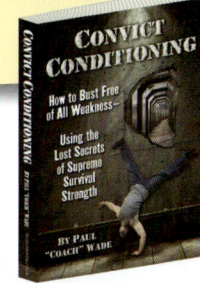

www.dragondoor.com
800·899·5111

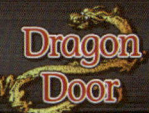

Order *Convict Conditioning* online:
www.dragondoor.com/B41

The Experts Give High Praise to Convict Conditioning 2

"Coach Paul Wade has outdone himself. His first book *Convict Conditioning* is to my mind THE BEST book ever written on bodyweight conditioning. Hands down. Now, with the sequel *Convict Conditioning 2*, Coach Wade takes us even deeper into the subtle nuances of training with the ultimate resistance tool: our bodies.

In plain English, but with an amazing understanding of anatomy, physiology, kinesiology and, go figure, psychology, Coach Wade explains very simply how to work the smaller but just as important areas of the body such as the hands and forearms, neck and calves and obliques in serious functional ways.

His minimalist approach to exercise belies the complexity of his system and the deep insight into exactly how the body works and the best way to get from A to Z in the shortest time possible.

I got the best advice on how to strengthen the hard-to-reach extensors of the hand right away from this exercise Master I have ever seen. It's so simple but so completely functional I can't believe no one else has thought of it yet. Just glad he figured it out for me.

Paul teaches us how to strengthen our bodies with the simplest of movements while at the same time balancing our structures in the same way: simple exercises that work the whole body.

And just as simply as he did with his first book. His novel approach to stretching and mobility training is brilliant and fresh as well as his take on recovery and healing from injury. Sprinkled throughout the entire book are too-many-to-count insights and advice from a man who has come to his knowledge the hard way and knows exactly of what he speaks.

This book is, as was his first, an amazing journey into the history of physical culture disguised as a book on calisthenics. But the thing that Coach Wade does better than any before him is his unbelievable progressions on EVERY EXERCISE and stretch! He breaks things down and tells us EXACTLY how to proceed to get to whatever level of strength and development we want. AND gives us the exact metrics we need to know when to go to the next level.

Adding in completely practical and immediately useful insights into nutrition and the mindset necessary to deal not only with training but with life, makes this book a classic that will stand the test of time.

Bravo Coach Wade, Bravo." —**Mark Reifkind**, Master RKC, author of *Mastering the HardStyle Kettlebell Swing*

"The overriding principle of *Convict Conditioning 2* is 'little equipment-big rewards'. For the athlete in the throwing and fighting arts, the section on Lateral Chain Training, Capturing the Flag, is a unique and perhaps singular approach to training the obliques and the whole family of side muscles. This section stood out to me as ground breaking and well worth the time and energy by anyone to review and attempt to complete. Literally, this is a new approach to lateral chain training that is well beyond sidebends and suitcase deadlifts.

The author's review of passive stretching reflects the experience of many of us in the field. But, his solution might be the reason I am going to recommend this work for everyone: The Trifecta. This section covers what the author calls The Functional Triad and gives a series of simple progressions to three holds that promise to oil your joints. It's yoga for the strength athlete and supports the material one would find, for example, in Pavel's *Loaded Stretching*.

I didn't expect to like this book, but I come away from it practically insisting that everyone read it. It is a strongman book mixed with yoga mixed with street smarts. I wanted to hate it, but I love it."
—**Dan John**, author of *Don't Let Go* and co-author of *Easy Strength*

"*Convict Conditioning* is one of the most influential books I ever got my hands on. *Convict Conditioning 2* took my training and outlook on the power of bodyweight training to the 10th degree—from strengthening the smallest muscles in a maximal manner, all the way to using bodyweight training as a means of healing injuries that pile up from over 22 years of aggressive lifting.

I've used both *Convict Conditioning* and *Convict Conditioning 2* on myself and with my athletes. Without either of these books I can easily say that these boys would not be the BEASTS they are today. Without a doubt *Convict Conditioning 2* will blow you away and inspire and educate you to take bodyweight training to a whole NEW level."
—**Zach Even-Esh**, Underground Strength Coach

Convict Conditioning 2
Advanced Prison Training Tactics for Muscle Gain, Fat Loss and Bulletproof Joints
By Paul "Coach" Wade
#B59 $39.95
Paperback 8.5 x 11 354 pages
261 photos, charts and illustrations

www.dragondoor.com
1·800·899·5111

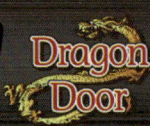

Order Convict Conditioning 2 online:
www.dragondoor.com/B59

CONVICT CONDITIONING 2
— TABLE OF CONTENTS —

Foreword
The Many Roads to Strength by Brooks Kubik

Opening Salvo: *Chewing Bubblegum and Kicking Ass*

1. Introduction: *Put Yourself Behind Bars*

PART I: SHOTGUN MUSCLE

Hands and Forearms

2: Iron Hands and Forearms: *Ultimate Strength —with Just Two Techniques*

3: The Hang Progressions: *A Vice-Like Bodyweight Grip Course*

4: Advanced Grip Torture: *Explosive Power + Titanium Fingers*

5: Fingertip Pushups: *Keeping Hand Strength Balanced*

6: Forearms into Firearms: *Hand Strength: A Summary and a Challenge*

Lateral Chain

7: Lateral Chain Training: *Capturing the Flag*

8: The Clutch Flag: *In Eight Easy Steps*

9: The Press Flag: *In Eight Not-So-Easy Steps*

Neck and Calves

10: Bulldog Neck: *Bulletproof Your Weakest Link*

11. Calf Training: *Ultimate Lower Legs—No Machines Necessary*

PART II: BULLETPROOF JOINTS

12. Tension-Flexibility: *The Lost Art of Joint Training*

13: Stretching—the Prison Take: *Flexibility, Mobility, Control*

14. The Trifecta: *Your "Secret Weapon" for Mobilizing Stiff, Battle-Scarred Physiques—for Life*

15: The Bridge Hold Progressions: *The Ultimate Prehab/Rehab Technique*

16: The L-Hold Progressions: *Cure Bad Hips and Low Back—Inside-Out*

17: Twist Progressions: *Unleash Your Functional Triad*

PART III: WISDOM FROM CELLBLOCK G

18. Doing Time Right: *Living the Straight Edge*

19. The Prison Diet: *Nutrition and Fat Loss Behind Bars*

20. Mendin' Up: *The 8 Laws of Healing*

21. The Mind: *Escaping the True Prison*

!BONUS CHAPTER!

Pumpin' Iron in Prison: *Myths, Muscle and Misconceptions*

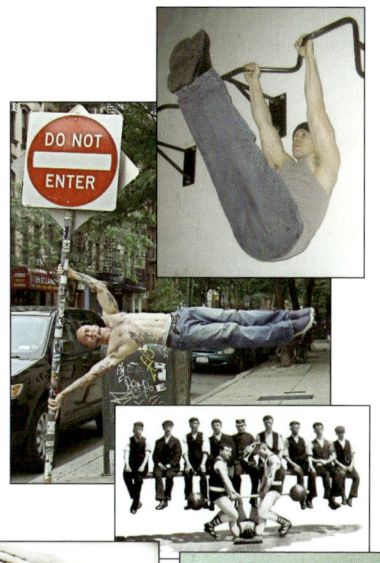

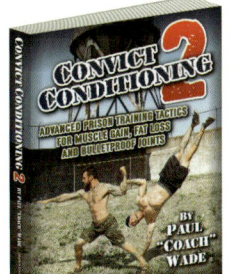

Convict Conditioning 2
Advanced Prison Training Tactics for Muscle Gain, Fat Loss and Bulletproof Joints

By Paul "Coach" Wade
#B59 $39.95

Paperback 8.5 x 11   354 pages
261 photos, charts and illustrations

www.dragondoor.com
800-899-5111

Order Convict Conditioning 2 online:
www.dragondoor.com/B59

GET DYNAMIC, CHISELLED, POWER-JACK LEGS AND DEVELOP EXPLOSIVE LOWER-BODY STRENGTH—WITH PAUL "COACH" WADE'S ULTIMATE BODYWEIGHT SQUAT COURSE

COMPLEX MADE SIMPLE

Having read both *Convict Conditioning* and *Convict Conditioning 2*, the complementary DVD series is an excellent translation of the big six movement progressions into a simple to follow DVD. The demonstration of movement progression through the 10 levels is well described and easy to follow. As a Physical Therapist it is a very useful way to teach safe progressions to patients/clients and other professionals. I have already used Volume I (the push up progression) to teach high school strength coaches how to safely progress athletes with pressing activity and look forward to using volume 2 with these same coaches. I think anyone who studies movement realizes very few athletes can properly squat with two legs, let alone one. You will not find an easier way to teach the squat. Well done again Paul. Look forward to the rest of the series."
—Andrew Marchesi PT/MPT, FAFS, Scottsdale, AZ

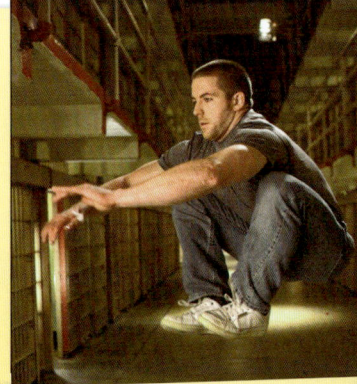

NAVY SEAL ON THE ROAD

"My whole team uses it. We can work out effectively anywhere and I mean anywhere!"—Tyler Archer, Navy

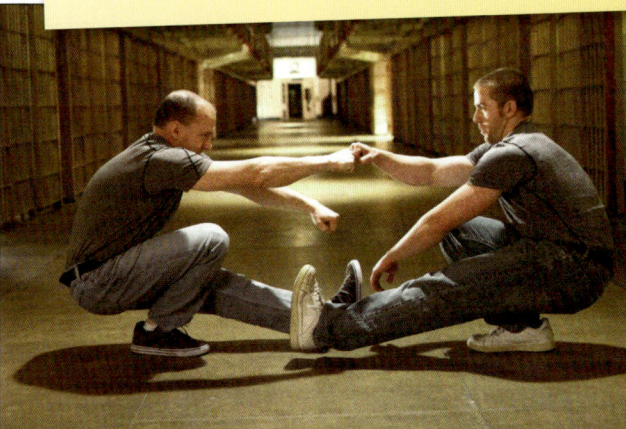

Convict Conditioning
Volume 2: The Ultimate Bodyweight Squat Course
By Paul "Coach" Wade featuring Brett Jones and Max Shank
#DV084 $69.95
DVD 56 minutes with full color Companion Manual, 88 pages

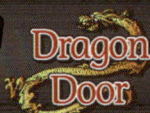

www.dragondoor.com
1·800·899·5111

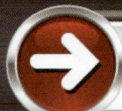

Order CC Ultimate Squat online:
www.dragondoor.com/DV084

Get a Rock-Hard, Brutishly Powerful Upper Frame and Achieve Elite-Level Strength— With Paul "Coach" Wade's
Prison-Style Pushup Program

Paul Wade's *Convict Conditioning* system represents the ultimate distillation of hardcore prison bodyweight training's most powerful methods. What works was kept. What didn't, was slashed away. When your life is on the line, you're not going to mess with less than the absolute best. Many of these older, very potent solitary training systems have been on the verge of dying, as convicts begin to gain access to weights, and modern "bodybuilding thinking" floods into the prisons. Thanks to Paul Wade, these ultimate strength survival secrets have been saved for posterity. And for you…

Filmed entirely—and so appropriately— on **"The Rock"**, Wade's *Convict Conditioning Prison Pushup Series* explodes out of the cellblock to teach you in absolute detail how to progress from the ease of a simple wall pushup—to the stunning "1-in-10,000" achievement of the prison-style one-arm pushup. Ten progressive steps guide you to pushup mastery. Do it—and become a Pushup God.

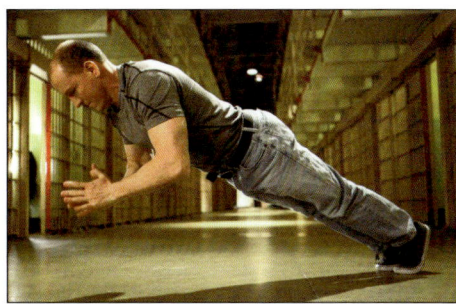

Awesome Resource for Coaches & Strength Devotees

"I am using this manual and DVD not just for my own training, but for the training of my athletes. It shocks and amazes me how varsity high school athletes can NOT perform a solid push up.... not even 1! Getting them to perform a perfect push up requires regressions, progressions, dialing in the little cues that teach them to generate tension and proper body alignment, ALL of which carry over to other exercises.

This manual is an awesome resource for Coaches. It can & should be used to educate those you train as well as shared with your staff. For those who have a love for strength, you will respect all the details given for each and every push up progression and you will use them and apply them.

As a Strength devotee for over 2 decades, I've been through the grinder with free weights and injuries, push ups are something **I KNOW** I'll be doing for the rest of my life which is why I RESPECT this course so much!

The lay out of this manual and DVD are also BIG time impressive, the old school look and feel fires me up and makes me wanna attack these push ups!"
—Zach Even-Esh, Manasquan, NJ

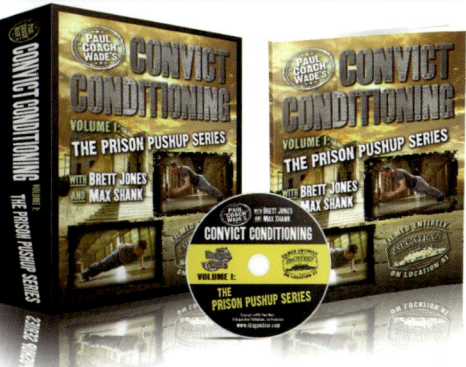

Convict Conditioning
Volume 1: The Prison Pushup Series
By Paul "Coach" Wade featuring Brett Jones and Max Shank
#DV083 $69.95
DVD 59 minutes with full color Companion Manual, 88 pages

www.dragondoor.com
800-899-5111

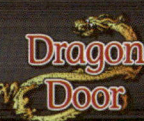

Order CC Prison Pushup online:
www.dragondoor.com/DV087

Demonic Abs Are a Man's Best Friend—Discover How to Seize a Six-Pack from Hell and OWN the World...
Leg Raises

Paul Wade's *Convict Conditioning 3, Leg Raises: Six Pack from Hell* teaches you in absolute detail how to progress from the ease of a simple Knee Tuck—to the magnificent, "1-in-1,000" achievement of the Hanging Straight Leg Raise. Ten progressive steps guide you to inevitable mastery of this ultimate abs exercise. Do it, seize the knowledge—but beware—the Gods will be jealous!

This home-study course in ultimate survival strength comes replete with bonus material not available in **Paul Wade's** original *Convict Conditioning* book—and numerous key training tips that refine and expand on the original program.

Prowl through the heavily and gorgeously-illustrated 80-plus-page manual and devour the entire film script at your animal leisure. Digest the brilliant, precise photographs and reinforce the raw benefits you absorbed from the DVD.

Paul Wade adds a bonus **Ten Commandments for Perfect Bodyweight Squats**—which is worth the price of admission alone. And there's the additional bonus of **4 major Variant drills** to add explosivity, fun and super-strength to your core practice.

Whatever you are looking for when murdering your abs—be it a fist-breaking, rock-like shield of impenetrable muscle, an uglier-is-more-beautiful set of rippling abdominal ridges, or a monstrous injection of lifting power—it's yours for the progressive taking with *Convict Conditioning, Volume 3, Leg Raises: Six Pack from Hell*

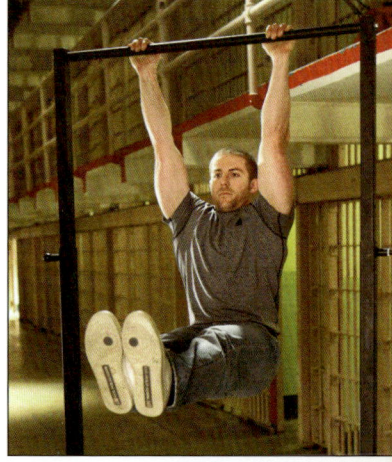

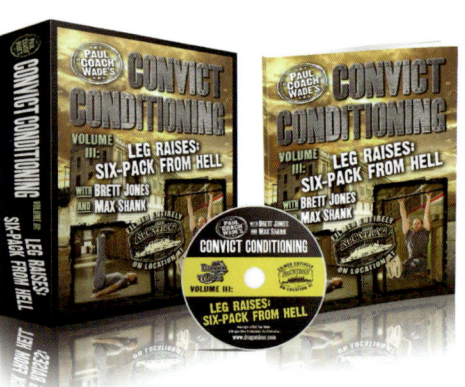

Convict Conditioning
Volume 3: Leg Raises Six Pack from Hell
By Paul "Coach" Wade featuring Brett Jones and Max Shank
#DV085 $59.95
DVD 57 minutes with full color Companion Manual, 82 pages

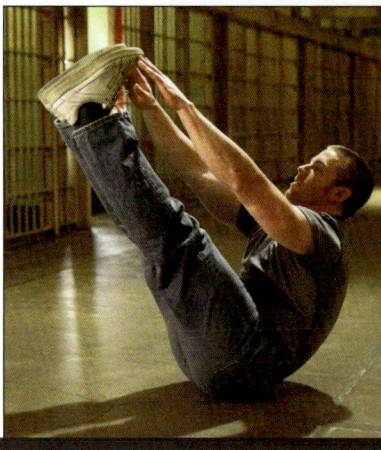

www.dragondoor.com
1•800•899•5111

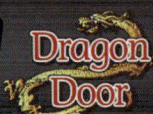

Order CC Ultimate Squat online:
www.dragondoor.com/DV085

Erect Twin Pythons of Coiled Beef Up Your Spine and Develop Extreme, Explosive Resilience—With the Dynamic Power and Flexible Strength of
ADVANCED BRIDGING

Paul Wade's *Convict Conditioning* system represents the ultimate distillation of hardcore prison bodyweight training's most powerful methods. What works was kept. What didn't, was slashed away. When your life is on the line, you're not going to mess with less than the absolute best. Many of these older, very potent solitary training systems have been on the verge of dying, as convicts begin to gain access to weights, and modern "bodybuilding thinking" floods into the prisons. Thanks to Paul Wade, these ultimate strength survival secrets have been saved for posterity. And for you…

Filmed entirely—and so appropriately— on **"The Rock"**, **Wade's** *Convict Conditioning Volume 4, Advanced Bridging: Forging an Iron Spine* explodes out of the cellblock to teach you in absolute detail how to progress from the relative ease of a Short Bridge—to the stunning, "1-in-1,000" achievement of the Stand-to-Stand Bridge. Ten progressive steps guide you to inevitable mastery of this ultimate exercise for an unbreakable back.

This home-study course in ultimate survival strength comes replete with bonus material not available in **Paul Wade's** original *Convict Conditioning* book—and numerous key training tips that refine and expand on the original program.

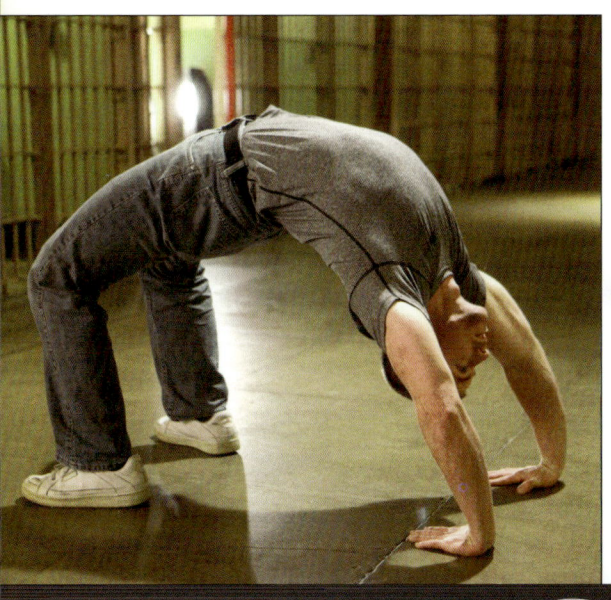
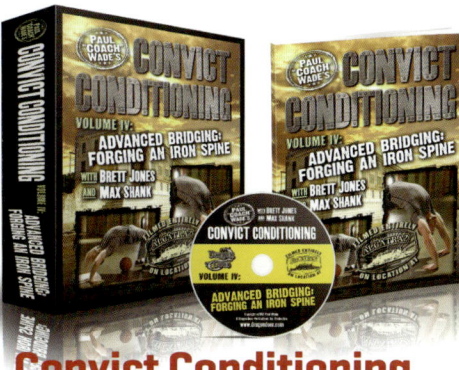

Convict Conditioning
Volume 4: Advanced Bridging: Forging an Iron Spine
By Paul "Coach" Wade featuring Brett Jones and Max Shank
#DV087 $59.95
DVD 59 minutes with full color Companion Manual, 88 pages

www.dragondoor.com
800·899·5111

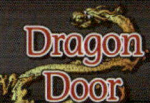

Order CC Prison Pushup online:
www.dragondoor.com/DV087

1·800·899·5111
24 HOURS A DAY
FAX YOUR ORDER (866) 280-7619

ORDERING INFORMATION

Customer Service Questions? Please call us between 9:00am– 11:00pm EST Monday to Friday at 1-800-899-5111. Local and foreign customers call 214-258-0134 for orders and customer service us, and please let us know why you were dissatisfied—it will help us to provide better products and services in the future. *Shipping and handling fees are non-refundable.*

100% One-Year Risk-Free Guarantee. If you are not completely satisfied with any product—we'll be happy to give you a prompt exchange, credit, or refund, as you wish. Simply return your purchase to

Telephone Orders For faster service you may place your orders by calling Toll Free 24 hours a day, 7 days a week, 365 days per year. When you call, please have your credit card ready.

Complete and mail with full payment to: Dragon Door Publications, 5 County Road B East, Suite 3, Little Canada, MN 55117

Please print clearly
Sold To: A

Name _____
Street _____
City _____
State _____ Zip _____
Day phone*_____
* Important for clarifying questions on orders

Please print clearly
SHIP TO: *(Street address for delivery)* B

Name _____
Street _____
City _____
State _____ Zip _____
Email _____

Warning to foreign customers:
The Customs in your country may or may not tax or otherwise charge you an additional fee for goods you receive. Dragon Door Publications is charging you only for U.S. handling and international shipping. Dragon Door Publications is in no way responsible for any additional fee levied by Customs, the carrier or any other entity.

ITEM #	QTY.	ITEM DESCRIPTION	ITEM PRICE	A OR B	TOTAL

HANDLING AND SHIPPING CHARGES— FOR MAIL ORDERS ONLY
Phone orders–your Dragon Door representative will give you the exact price
Website orders–shipping and handling will display automatically
Total Amount of Order Add (Excludes kettlebells and kettlebell kits):

$00.00 to 29.99	Add $7.30	100.00 to 129.99	Add
$30.00 to 49.99	Add $8.35	$15.70	
$50.00 to 69.99	Add $9.45	130.00 to 169.99	Add
$70.00 to 99.99	Add $12.55	$7.80	
		170.00 to 199.99	Add $19.90

Canada and Mexico double the charges. All other countries triple the charges.

Total of Goods	
Shipping Charges	
Rush Charges	
Kettlebell Shipping Charges	
TX residents add 8.25% sales tax	
MN residents add 7.125% sales tax	
TOTAL ENCLOSED	

Warning!
This may be the last issue of the catalog you receive.

If we rented your name, or you haven't ordered in the last two years you may not hear from us again. If you wish to stay informed about products and services that can make a difference to your health and well-being, please indicate below.

Name _____
Address _____
City _____ State ____ Zip ____
Phone _____

Do You Have A Friend Who'd Like To Receive This Catalog?

We would be happy to send your friend a free copy. Make sure to print and complete in full:

Name _____
Address _____
City _____ State ____ Zip ____

METHOD OF PAYMENT ❏ CHECK ❏ M.O. ❏ MASTERCARD ❏ VISA ❏ DISCOVER ❏ AMEX
Account No. (Please indicate all numbers on your credit card) EXPIRATION DATE   CCV

☐☐☐☐ ☐☐☐☐ ☐☐☐☐ ☐☐☐☐   ☐☐/☐☐   ☐☐☐

Day Phone: ( ) _____
Signature: _____ **Date:** _____

NOTE: *We ship best method available for your delivery address. Foreign orders are sent by air. Credit card or International M.O. only.* For **RUSH** *processing of your order, add an additional $10.00 per address. Available on money order & charge card orders only.*

Errors and omissions excepted. Prices subject to change without notice.

1·800·899·5111
24 HOURS A DAY
FAX YOUR ORDER (866) 280-7619

  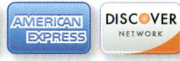

ORDERING INFORMATION

Customer Service Questions? Please call us between 9:00am– 11:00pm EST Monday to Friday at 1-800-899-5111. Local and foreign customers call 214-258-0134 for orders and customer service

100% One-Year Risk-Free Guarantee. If you are not completely satisfied with any product—we'll be happy to give you a prompt exchange, credit, or refund, as you wish. Simply return your purchase to us, and please let us know why you were dissatisfied—it will help us to provide better products and services in the future. *Shipping and handling fees are non-refundable.*

Telephone Orders For faster service you may place your orders by calling Toll Free 24 hours a day, 7 days a week, 365 days per year. When you call, please have your credit card ready.

Complete and mail with full payment to: Dragon Door Publications, 5 County Road B East, Suite 3, Little Canada, MN 55117

Please print clearly

Sold To: A

Name _____

Street _____

City _____

State _____ Zip _____

Day phone* _____
*Important for clarifying questions on orders

Please print clearly

SHIP TO: (Street address for delivery) B

Name _____

Street _____

City _____

State _____ Zip _____

Email _____

Warning to foreign customers:

The Customs in your country may or may not tax or otherwise charge you an additional fee for goods you receive. Dragon Door Publications is charging you only for U.S. handling and international shipping. Dragon Door Publications is in no way responsible for any additional fees levied by Customs, the carrier or any other entity.

Warning! This may be the last issue of the catalog you receive.

If we rented your name, or you haven't ordered in the last two years you may not hear from us again. If you wish to stay informed about products and services that can make a difference to your health and well-being, please indicate below.

Name _____

Address _____

City _____ State _____ Zip _____

Phone _____

Do You Have A Friend Who'd Like To Receive This Catalog?

We would be happy to send your friend a free copy. Make sure to print and complete in full:

Name _____

Address _____

City _____ State _____ Zip _____

Item #	Qty.	Item Description	Item Price	A or B	Total

HANDLING AND SHIPPING CHARGES— FOR MAIL ORDERS ONLY

Phone orders–your Dragon Door representative will give you the exact price
Website orders–shipping and handling will display automatically
Total Amount of Order Add **(Excludes kettlebells and kettlebell kits):**

$0.00 to 29.99	Add $7.30	$100.00 to 129.99 Add
$0.00 to 49.99	Add $8.35	$15.70
$0.00 to 69.99	Add $9.40	$130.00 to 169.99 Add
$0.00 to 99.99	Add $12.55	$7.80
		$170.00 to 199.99 Add $19.90

Canada and Mexico double the charges, All other countries triple the charges.

Total of Goods	
Shipping Charges	
Rush Charges	
Kettlebell Shipping Charges	
TX residents add 8.25% sales tax	
MN residents add 7.125% sales tax	
TOTAL ENCLOSED	

METHOD OF PAYMENT ☐ Check ☐ M.O. ☐ Mastercard ☐ Visa ☐ Discover ☐ Amex

Account No. (Please indicate all numbers on your credit card)   EXPIRATION DATE   CCV

☐☐☐☐ ☐☐☐☐ ☐☐☐☐ ☐☐☐☐   ☐☐/☐☐   ☐☐☐

Phone: ( ) _____

Signature: _____ Date: _____

*We ship best method available for your delivery address. Foreign orders are sent by air. Credit card or International M.O. only. For **RUSH** processing of your order, add an additional $10.00 per address. Available on money order & charge card orders only.

Errors and omissions excepted. Prices subject to change without notice.*